The Nurses' Handbook
of Complementary Therapies

For Churchill Livingstone

Commissioning editor: Inta Ozols
Project editor: Dinah Thom
Project manager: Valerie Burgess
Project controller: Nicola Haig/Pat Miller
Designer: Judith Wright
Sales promotion executive: Hilary Brown

The Nurses' Handbook of Complementary Therapies

Edited by

Denise F. Rankin-Box BA (Hons) RGN DipTD CertEd
Senior Lecturer in Nursing and Health Studies and Director, Centre for
Complementary Medicine, North West Faculty of ASS, School of Nursing and
Health Studies, Stockport College of Further and Higher Education, Stockport, UK

Foreword by

Christine Hancock
General Secretary, Royal College of Nursing, London, UK

CHURCHILL LIVINGSTONE
EDINBURGH LONDON MADRID MELBOURNE NEW YORK AND TOKYO 1995

CHURCHILL LIVINGSTONE
Medical Division of Longman Group Limited

Distributed in the United States of America by Churchill Livingstone Inc., 650
Avenue of the Americas, New York, N.Y. 10011, and by associated companies,
branches and representatives throughout the world.

First published 1995

ISBN 0 443 051801

British Library Cataloguing in Publication Data
A catalogue record for this book is available from the British Library.

Library of Congress Cataloging in Publication Data
A catalog record for the book is available from the Library of Congress.

The
publisher's
policy is to use
**paper manufactured
from sustainable forests**

Produced through Longman Malaysia

Contents

Contributors

Kenneth Atherton FSBioMed BRCP (ClassicalHom) SRN A&ECert DNCert OpThCert EAV&VegaCert (West Germany) AssocFacHom (Royal London Homoeopathic Hospital)
Lecturer in Homoeopathic Medicine to nurses and health professionals, University College, Stockport (University accredited course); Guest Lecturer, Complementary and Homoeopathic Medicine, Faculty of Nursing , University of Liverpool; Practical Demonstrator in Homoeopathy to fifth year medical students and final year student nurses

David Bray DC (USA)
Founder Member/former Information Officer, International Stress Management Association, UK; Member, Association of Applied Psychophysiology and Biofeedback, USA; Trustee, Russian International Academy of Science, Moscow

Helen Busby MSc MNIMH
Freelance Researcher and Consultant Medical Herbalist

Clare Byrne RGN BA(Hons) FETC DPSN
Clinical Research Facilitator, Nursing Development Unit, Royal Liverpool University Hospital, Liverpool

Dorothy Crowther RGN RCNT RNT FRCN
Chief Executive, Wirral Holistic Care Services, St Catherine's Hospital, Birkenhead, Wirral

Stephanie Downey RGN BA(Hons) BAc
Acupuncturist, Brighton Acupuncture Clinic, Brighton

Elizabeth Evans MA BA Cert Cains Cert Ed RGN
Lecturer in Sociology and Counselling, Centre for Complementary Medicine, North West Faculty of ASS, School of Nursing and Health Studies, Stockport College of Further and Higher Education, Stockport

Pamela Griffiths RGN BA ONC RCNT RNT Cert Ed
Nurse Teacher, South East Wales Institute of Nursing and Midwifery, Cardiff Royal Infirmary, Cardiff

Carol Horrigan MSc SRN RCNT DipN PGCEA RNT
Lecturer in Complementary Therapies, Royal College of Nursing, London

Maxine L. V-T. McVey RN
Senior Sister, St Mark's Hospital, London

Jane Mallett BSc MSc RGN
Research and Practice Development Co-ordinator, The Royal Marsden NHS Trust, London

Denise F. Rankin-Box BA (Hons) RGN DipTD CertEd
Senior Lecturer in Nursing and Health Studies and Director, Centre for Complementary Medicine, North West Faculty of ASS, School of Nursing and Health Studies, Stockport College of Further and Higher Education, Stockport

Lynne Ryman RGN ONC NFSH
Relaxation Therapist, Rehabilitation Unit, Royal Marsden Hospital, London

Jean Sayre-Adams MA RN(US)
Director and Senior Lecturer, Didsbury Trust, Litton, Near Bath

Caroline Stevensen BA (Hons) RGN MRSS IFA Master Iridologist
Macmillan Nurse Specialist, Royal London Homoeopathic Hospital NHS Trust, London

Foreword

This handbook of complementary therapy for nurses is both timely and interesting. It is a valuable resource for nurses who are actively involved in using complementary therapy, and those who are interested in expanding their practice to offer greater choice to patients and clients.

In recent years, there has been growing pressure on nurses to prove their value in terms of their cost effectiveness and their contribution to patient well being. Nurses have accepted this challenge, proving that qualified nursing care not only helps people to get better quicker, but in the long term, it actually costs less.

One of the most important aspects of nursing's contribution is the added value it brings to the health care team. Nurses bring a new dimension to care, increasing the variety as well as the volume and the quality of care available.

Based on a growing confidence of this value, nurses everywhere are pushing at the boundaries of care to find innovative ways of solving long standing problems. The increased use and greater understanding of complementary therapies provides a good example of this.

Nurses understand the importance of basing their practice on experience and research. Nursing research enables them to ensure that innovative practice really does enhance the quality of care that patients receive. At the same time, for nursing to continue to develop as a flourishing, autonomous, practice – based discipline, it must be replenished and strengthened by the new knowledge and new insights derived from research.

Nurses also understand that changing the way things are done can cause its own difficulties. Introducing complementary therapies into practice requires a cautious and sensitive approach with colleagues and patients alike.

Thus, the handbook's exploration of research issues and how to choose and manage a therapy is invaluable.

The handbook includes a comprehensive introduction to many of the therapies used by nurses today and the way in which they are being applied in a range of settings.

As such, the handbook is an excellent working guide, and a constructive tool in the wider and continuing debate on the value of nursing.

London 1995   Christine Hancock

Preface

Increasing interest in the use of complementary therapies within nursing practice means that there will inevitably be a plethora of texts appearing on the market. As more books appear promoting disparate and more unusual approaches to health care, the practical indications for the use of a therapy by nurses may unwittingly be overlooked in the desire to try to help clients in whatever way seems most appropriate.

Such an approach is perhaps only part of the therapeutic strategy. These days, reading about a therapy and indeed training in one may not be sufficient to enable you to practise in the health care setting. With this in mind, the first section of this handbook identifies key areas that nurses should consider when attempting to successfully integrate complementary therapies into health care practice. These include choosing a therapy, managing change in the workplace, policy development and research issues to be aware of when critically evaluating or planning research studies.

Section 2 of the handbook is designed as a guide to provide nurses with a concise, substantiated introduction to the complementary therapies most commonly used in nursing practice today. Throughout the text the implications for nursing practice are paramount, and each therapy identifies both indications and contraindications for use.

This book is presented as a guide to key issues that are central in the debate concerning complementary therapies in nursing practice today. As such it does not validate any names, addresses or courses mentioned in the text, nor is it a DIY manual. The intention is to facilitate your future studies and research in this field. Any suggestions from readers concerning topics to be included in the next handbook would be greatly appreciated.

A principal aim of this book is that it should be a working text — something you can carry around, use as an easy reference guide, with at-a-glance boxes highlighting key issues and with some blank pages at the back for your own notes. I hope we have achieved this — if it becomes dog-eared and full of comments and notes, with the telephone numbers of your ethical committee, policy development or finance officers and so on then it has become a working text. Even if you choose not to use it in this way, I hope it serves to stimulate and promote professional practice in the use of innovative forms of therapeutic care.

Prestbury 1995   D. F. R-B.

Acknowledgements

Grateful thanks are extended to the Royal College of Nursing for permission to use Complementary Therapy documents developed by the Complementary Therapies in Nursing Forum Steering Group. Thanks also to all the contributors for their time, commitment and support in this endeavour — it was greatly appreciated. Special thanks to my husband Ian for his continued support and for providing the time and space for me to complete the manuscript; also to our daughters Carla and Felicity who have in their own unique ways shown me different ways of perceiving and asking questions about the world. I am also grateful to Maureen Eccleston for her unflagging professional and personal encouragement in promoting complementary therapies in nursing practice.

1 Introduction

Denise Rankin-Box

'It is one of the commonest of mistakes to consider that the limit of our power of perception is also the limit of all there is to perceive' C. W. Leadbeater

Complementary therapies in health care are not new. The use of herbs, oils, laying on of hands or the treatment of forms of energy within the human body appear to have existed in some form or another for thousands of years. Complementary therapies do not represent a rediscovery of therapeutic forms of healing — peoples in tribes and multifarious cultures around the world have continued to use natural forms of health care and ritualized approaches to healing over the centuries. Indeed there has never been a time when many of the therapies described in this handbook have not been in existence somewhere in human history. However, the social recognition afforded to certain therapies and reliance placed upon their efficacy appears to have shifted over time.

Social trends and cultural change similarly influence a person's health care beliefs. As a result, some health care practices such as herbalism or healing have been the object of ridicule and persecution during certain periods of social history. Perhaps current health care trends demanding choice in health care treatment are simply social trends and a response to consumer desire in the search for the 'panacea for all ills'.

Interestingly the shift towards individualized forms of health care is not only occurring in one small area of western society but, according to the British Medical Association (BMA), a number of indicators suggests that there has been an increase in the use of non-conventional therapies not only in the UK but also in the US and in Europe (BMA 1993). Even allowing for greater communication across nations using current technology it is not easy to explain the current explosion of interest in the use of complementary medicine in health care. In part, there may be disillusionment with the perceived limitations of reductionist forms of medicine and the apparent failure to treat and/ or cure chronic illness and catastrophic disease such as cancer or AIDS.

To some extent, disquiet focusing upon the failures of modern medicine is a little misplaced. Whilst a number of medical 'break-throughs' might appear to be a little like taking a sledgehammer to crack a nut, many other developments have undoubtedly wrought modern-day miracles in the management of illness. Ironically, it could be that current systems of medical practice have been hoisted by their own petard — the very successes enhancing health and ex-tending longevity have given birth to a new generation of illnesses and dilemmas previously limited by shorter lifespans.

Additionally, the successful use of preventive medicine and enhanced quality of health in the West has resulted in an increasingly critical reflection of the way in which health and illness is perceived and care meted out when treating disorders. There is growing recognition of the interplay between mind and body upon the state of an indivi-dual's health and wellbeing. This has resulted in the recognition of the process of care as well as the outcome and the role of the therapeutic relationship in facilitating the healing process.

Within nursing practice the nature of care provided for a client is dependent upon some form of therapeutic relationship. This was described by Hockey 'as the practice of those nursing activities which have a healing effect or those which result in a movement towards health or wellness' (Hockey 1991). The use of complementary therapies within nursing practice not only builds upon this approach to care but seeks to utilize nursing practice in a specific way — to proactively negotiate and facilitate the healing process using specific therapeutic procedures. Such an approach is challenging and innovative since it obviates generalistic approaches to current models of nursing laying claim to highly individualized systems of health care based upon a case-load approach.

ABOUT THIS BOOK

Although there has been a great expansion of interest, research and publishing in the field of complementary medicine there has been little attempt to highlight a number of practical issues associated with the formal development and integration of complementary therapies within the workplace. Additionally, whilst many books testify to the benefits of specific therapies, in general, texts do not focus upon the use and implications certain therapies may have with immuno-compromised clients and so indications and contraindications of use are not clearly presented. The aim of this book was to try to go some way to resolving these dilemmas for nurses wishing to include certain therapies in nursing practice.

The topics and therapies selected for inclusion were those that nurses had expressed an interest in, to me, and come not only from the UK but also the US, Canada, Israel and Australia. Knowing about therapies is not enough; for this approach to become successfully integrated into mainstream nursing practice, protocol development, managing change and research awareness are essential.

The aim was to develop a user-friendly handbook that nurses could carry around with them; small enough to keep in a pocket and designed in such a way as to provide easy access to any part of the handbook. I hope we have gone some way to meeting this need.

As nursing practice continues to evolve, reflect and dynamically shape health care trends in society, so more therapies and associated administrative issues will come to the fore and a second handbook will become necessary. Clearly developments in this field of care should not be perceived as exclusive to nursing care. Close collaboration across the professional health care spectrum can only serve to promote and integrate complementary medicine within orthodox practice. Additionally, initiating professional debate concerning treatment efficacy, the substantive base of certain therapies and the issues of educational competence reinforces the proactive stance that the nursing profession is willing to adopt in order to provide a therapeutic partnership in care.

As we begin to question current perceptions of health and illness we should also begin to ask questions about the general way in which we perceive these. Indeed, as Reilly and Taylor suggest 'proof is more often demanded than defined' (Reilly & Taylor 1993).

REFERENCES

BMA 1993 Complementary medicine: new approaches to good practice. British Medical Association, Oxford University Press, Oxford
Hockey L 1991 In: McMahon R, Pearson A (eds) Nursing as therapy. Chapman and Hall, London, p X
Reilly D, Taylor M 1993 Summary of methods and achievements. Developing Integrated Medicine. Complementary Therapies in Medicine 1 (supp): 6

SECTION 1

Introducing complementary therapies in the workplace

2 Choosing a therapy

Clare Byrne

INTRODUCTION

When considering the use of a therapy two principal issues arise — the selection of a therapy for personal treatment and consideration of selection of a therapy/course in which to train. These issues are addressed separately and guidelines to facilitate selection are presented.

Under common law in the UK anyone can set up as a practitioner (or trainer), and so an informed guide to the selection and use of a therapy is valuable.

In 1993, the British Medical Association (BMA) suggested that approximately 180 different therapies are practised in the UK. To date only osteopathy has obtained legislative power to sanction individuals guilty of malpractice. For many therapies, work continues towards developing and monitoring educational standards and practice competencies. Against this background, the selection of a therapy for personal or client use can be difficult.

When choosing a therapy for oneself or for a client group it is valuable to have a wider perspective of the different therapies:

- Many complementary therapies represent systems of medicine; for example, acupuncture, homoeopathy and herbalism. This is in contrast to treatments such as iridology, which is primarily a diagnostic tool, or biofeedback, massage and aromatherapy, which are primarily therapeutic (Pietroni 1990, Rankin-Box 1991).

- Some complementary therapies are derived from past cultural and social structures, such as the ancient Egyptian and Chinese civilizations. The approach taken to evaluating the effectiveness and suitability of such therapies may differ from that of orthodox scientific medical interventions. Stevensen (1992b) suggests that although the more physical, obvious and therefore measurable effects of a complementary therapy, may make it easier to evaluate scientifically, the patient's response is also important.

- Certain complementary therapies build upon the therapeutic relationship (McMahon and Pearson 1991); care covers not only the physical aspects of a person's condition but also the emotional, mental, psychological and spiritual dimensions.

CHOOSING A COMPLEMENTARY THERAPY WITHIN A HEALTH CARE SETTING

The following criteria for choice of therapy were identified by Wafer (1994) when exploring the introduction of complementary therapies into a busy unit for care of the elderly:

- The therapy could be used in everyday practice
- The therapy would complement interdisciplinary care
- The therapy could be realistically introduced
- The therapy should be non-invasive
- The therapy should provide relaxation and comfort.

Other authors such as Armstrong & Waldron (1991), Stevensen (1992a) and Burke & Sikora (1992) have also identified criteria for therapy selection in different clinical areas. Additional considerations are as follows:

- Who is the therapy for?
- Are research data available to substantiate the use of the therapy?
- Is a nurse able to provide the therapy or will the therapy be provided by a specialized practitioner?
- Is the therapy being used as part of a multidisciplinary health care team approach?
- What is the cost and who will pay if the therapy is not available on the NHS?
- What are the resource implications, e.g. time, space, training, materials?
- What are the legal implications of use of the therapy, including insurance and informed consent?

CONSUMER GUIDE

In 1993, the Royal College of Nursing issued a consumer checklist (developed by the Special Interest Group in Complementary Therapies in Nursing [CTINSIG]) for complementary therapies, to help patients or clients feel more confident about choosing a therapy. Some of the points they identified are listed below:

- What are the therapist's qualifications and how long was the training?
- Is the therapist a member of a recognized, registered body with codes of practice?
- Can the therapist provide the address and telephone number of this organization to check?
- Is the therapy available on the NHS?
- Can a GP delegate care to the therapist?
- Is this the most appropriate complementary therapy for the particular problem?
- Does the therapist send a letter to the GP advising of any treatment received?
- Can the patient/client claim for the therapy through a private health insurance scheme?
- Are the patient records confidential?
- What is the cost of the treatment?
- How many treatments will be needed (and therefore what is the total cost)?
- What insurance cover does the therapist have?

CHOOSING A COURSE

Carers, such as nurses, occupational therapists and physiotherapists, who have experienced the benefits of complementary therapies or who recognize their potential for enhancing their current therapeutic role often proceed to train in a therapy. In reply to constant requests from its members, the Royal College of Nursing, Department of Nursing Policy and Practice, published, in association with the CTINSIG, guidelines in 1992 called 'Choosing a complementary therapies course — what should you consider?'. These guidelines are outlined here. Whilst they are concerned with nursing, they could readily be used by other health care disciplines.

First, it is important to examine personal reasons for wanting to take a complementary therapy course. These might be:

- to use such therapies in conjunction with nursing skills

- to develop a new career
- to enhance self-awareness.

Then there are the obvious practical considerations:

- what qualifications are needed
- the length of the course
- how much the course costs (remember time is a cost)
- whether an employer will help fund the course
- if there is scope for development in the nurse's current area of work.

Some useful feedback can be got from other nurses who have undertaken a particular complementary therapies course. It is also helpful to visit the institution and speak to the trainers. (Note that correspondence courses are best avoided as they are often difficult to complete or validate.)

It is essential to determine if the course is validated by any examining bodies, whether there is accreditation, and what European Community regulations affect the therapy in question. Regarding course content and structure, check which of the following are included:

- supervised training practice
- anatomy and physiology
- practical examination
- theory examination
- supervised clinical practice
- counselling/communication and self-development skills
- support for the trainee therapist
- business skills.

Other questions to ask are:

- Does the course take an holistic approach?
- Support for the trainee therapist
- What are the qualifications of the teaching staff, and are they appropriate?
- How many will be in the class (what is the tutor/pupil ratio)?

Finally, a 'taster' weekend is a good way to get the feel of a course before making a commitment.

CHOOSING A PRACTITIONER

GP clinics, health centres

Since 1993 it has been possible to delegate NHS client care to complementary therapists. Many General Practice (GP) fundholders now employ complementary therapists in their health care team. The GP must, according to the medical code of conduct, retain overall responsibility.

Professional registering organizations

The professional organizations for the different therapies should be able to provide a list of local registered practitioners. The British Holistic Medical Association (BHMA) holds names and addresses for these professional organizations — see also the addresses listed at the back of this book.

Summary

Choosing a complementary therapy whether for personal use or to enhance the therapeutic role entails thorough investigation of potential benefits. It is important to evaluate critically the research data available. Knowledge of the various therapies can be developed through information gathering and personal experience at workshops. Additionally, there are practical considerations such as availability of a registered practitioner. When considering training, availability of validated courses, the approval of all members of the multidisciplinary team, and consideration of how to evaluate the effectiveness of the complementary therapy intervention must be taken into account.

Those who have used complementary therapies for themselves and for their client group usually recommend proceeding with caution. Consider why and whether a therapy is needed for a specific client group. Critically evaluate the potential benefits or contra-indications regarding the use of a therapy and objectively appraise the evidence underpinning a therapy and training programme offered.

REFERENCES

Armstrong F, Waldran R 1991 A complementary strategy. Nursing Times 87: 34–35
Burke C, Sikora K 1992 Cancer — the dual approach. Nursing Times 88: 62–66
Pietroni P 1990 The greening of medicine. Victor Gollancz, London
Rankin-Box D 1991 Proceed with caution. Nursing Times 87: 34–36
Stevensen C 1992a Appropriate therapies for nurses to practise. Nursing Standard 6: 51–52
Stevensen C 1992b Holistic power. Nursing Standard 88: 68–70
Wafer M 1994 Finding the formula to enhance care. Professional Nurse March: 414–417

FURTHER READING

McMahon R, Pearson A 1991 Nursing as therapy. Chapman and Hall, London
Rankin-Box D (ed) 1988 Complementary health therapies. A guide for nurses and the caring professions. Croom Helm, London
Rankin-Box D 1993 Innovations in practice: complementary therapies in nursing. Complementary Therapies in Medicine 2: 27–35

USEFUL ADDRESSES

British Holistic Medicine Association
179 Gloucester Place
London NW1 6DX

Centre for Complementary
Medicine (North West)
School of Nursing and Health
Studies
Stockport College of Further and
Higher Education
Wellington Road South
Stockport SK1 3UQ

Institute for Complementary
Medicine
PO Box 194
London SE16 IQ2

Research Council for
Complementary Medicine
60 Great Ormond Street
London
WC1N 3HR

Royal College of Nursing
20 Cavendish Square
London
W1M OAB

3 Managing change in the workplace

Denise Rankin-Box

'There is nothing permanent except change' Heraclitus (540–475 BC)

INTRODUCTION

There are a number of general issues associated with the introduction of complementary therapies into a clinical setting and these can be illustrated by some examples of general strategies of change. The examples provided here are not exhaustive but hopefully show how innovative approaches to health care may be implemented within the clinical setting.

When integrating complementary therapies in orthodox health care, the rate and direction of change in a particular setting can vary markedly. Some pioneers will encounter few problems, but they are perhaps in the minority. Many others will face seemingly insurmountable hurdles to changing practice or introducing a new approach. Some will identify the direction in which they wish to develop but fail to select an appropriate strategy to facilitate the change. This chapter looks at ways of easing the process of change.

CHANGE

Change is an inevitable aspect of daily life. However, as Toffler (1970) suggests, the rate of change has implications distinct from the direction of change. In the myriad organizational structures and institutions of today's society, rate and direction of change may not be well-matched. Frequently individuals or groups are exorted to take on board new ideas that have radical implications for their work. Varying rates of change across society or a profession can result in considerable stress or burnout as people attempt to adjust and adapt to unprecedented change (Moss Kanter 1984).

In the field of health care, organizations are under pressure to cut costs and yet improve services in the face of government regulation and the growth of cost-effective and profit-oriented hospital structures (Moss Kanter 1984). In the midst of the rapid change in many areas of health care there has been critical appraisal and reflection on the nature of nursing and the priorities and direction of health care delivery. Complementary approaches within health care represent one aspect of change that has been initiated mainly by nurses rather than management. In contrast to the seemingly impersonal organizational changes in health care, this approach gives greater priority to the needs of clients and their carers than to those of the organization. It reflects a radical change of direction in the philosophy of health care provision. Identifying the direction of change implies reflective acknowledgement that things have moved on; values have shifted and a restructuring of health care provision is required. Direction provides the vision for change. The rate at which such a change can be successfully implemented is influenced by issues associated with the management of change.

Wright (1989) suggests that nurses can be effective agents of change. Nursing can influence social and individual health and well-being, and Wright argues that if we believe our actions are utilitarian then there is a responsibility to ensure we control the delivery and quality of our service; this implies both individual and political commitment to change. Wright notes that because change produces individual stress related to a perceived lack of control, we must determine the nature and direction of change. A knowledge of the process of change is essential for the effective integration of complementary approaches to health care. It encourages nurses to be proactive in determining the course of the profession (Wright 1989), and to become masters not slaves of change (Moss Kanter 1983).

APPROACHES TO CHANGE

People differ in their ability to manage change (Dobson et al 1988). Some welcome change whilst others prefer more stable conditions. Thus, Gillies (1989) suggests that a well-planned strategy for change be developed. The selection of a particular model should take into account the situation and the beliefs, values and behaviour of the people who are to experience the change (Haffer 1986).

There are a number of models of change theory in the literature, such as Lewin 1953, Seifert & Clinebell 1969, Lippitt 1970. They highlight ways in which change may occur:

- Lewin (1953) suggests three phases — unfreezing, moving and then refreezing — a process by which an individual is encouraged to reflect critically upon current practice, new concepts are introduced and considered and finally the idea is adopted and change occurs creating another status quo.

■ Seifert & Clinebell (1969) and Lippitt (1970) adopt a problem-solving approach to the management of change involving diagnosis of a problem and subsequent steps taken to manage the process of change effectively.

The approach adopted depends on the environment in which the change is to be introduced. The steps listed here provide a general guide and build upon the stages identified by Lippitt (1970).

■ Recognize the need for change
■ Diagnose why
■ Team recognizes why
■ Team recognizes the need for change
■ Identify the aim
■ Consider alternate courses of action/practice
■ Set clear, achievable objectives
■ Reinforce positively when objectives are met by the team
■ Monitor and evaluate the process of change
■ Review and appraise.

STRATEGIES FOR CHANGE

There are three key strategies for change: power coercive, rational empirical and normative re-educative.

Power coercive. This assumes a 'top-down' approach to change. Underpinning the strategy is a belief that knowledge is power which can be used to achieve a desired outcome (Keyzer 1989). It is commonly associated with hierarchical systems of management.

Rational empirical. This assumes people are rational and self-interested and will view change positively, as long there are benefits (Bennis et al 1976). An example of the rational empirical approach is telling people that cigarette smoking is dangerous to health in order to alter smoking behaviour.

Normative re-educative. This is influenced by the perception a group or individual has of both the need for and value of change. Keyzer (1989) notes that this approach offers a means of drawing upon the organization's perceptions of the need for change as well as individual or group needs. It requires team participation in change and forms the basis for the belief that the process of change should build upon collaboration between the client and the agent of change.

A normative re-educative strategy is commonly considered the most effective stance to adopt for change. It facilitates a multidisciplinary approach to changing health care by the introduction of a complementary therapy.

KEY ISSUES TO BE AWARE OF WHEN MANAGING CHANGE

The introduction of an innovative approach to health care must be carefully planned before implementation. Where possible, a normative re-educative strategy will facilitate a multidisciplinary approach towards the introduction of a therapy within daily practice. Some common considerations for the introduction of complementary therapies in the work setting are listed next (adapted from Moss Kanter 1984 — an account of hurdles commonly encountered when attempting to manage change). They reflect concerns raised by many nurse practitioners attempting to introduce complementary therapies and holistic procedures to daily practice.

- **Loss of control**
  Attitudes to change are influenced by the extent to which people feel in control. Lack of control makes people feel powerless. Moss Kanter (1984) suggests 'it is powerlessness that corrupts — not power'. Individuals not in control may seek to undermine the process of change.
  Solution: Offer people choices and a sense of ownership over the change/selection of a therapy.

- **Excess uncertainty**
  Individuals resist change if they are not sure where the change will take them and what the long-term implications are.
  Solution: Divide any large-scale or radical change into small achievable steps to reduce the sense of risk or threat. Giving frequent information and updates can allay anxieties as well as providing a clear vision of overall change.

■ **Innovative therapies are different**
Rapid change can be exhausting because habits and rituals are upturned or removed. Learning new routines and patterns of care may make people feel they no longer know how to do their work — and this can be both stressful and draining.

Solution: Highlight the similarities between previous, familiar practices and new therapies. For instance, preparing a client for a massage, reflexology or aromatherapy treatment has similarities with, for example, preparation for blanket bathing, pressure care or other forms of physical care. By highlighting the familiar, the team are able to retain some habits and routines.

■ **Losing face**
In the enthusiasm of introducing something you are convinced is a better approach to nursing care, there is a danger that past actions may be perceived as 'not good enough' or 'wrong'.

Solution: Put past actions into context. Previous actions may have been excellent. However, times have changed and information and practices not readily available before may now be considered as potential ways in which to improve already high standards of care.

■ **Change is work**
Introducing change to the clinical setting takes considerable work. There is the inception and analysis of an idea, strategic planning, discussion, the process of implementation and finally evaluation of effectiveness.

Solution: Acknowledge this with the team. Be honest. Where possible, reward hard work to facilitate commitment to the change.

A crucial aspect of successful change is effective communication amongst the multidisciplinary team. When attempting to introduce complementary therapies into the clinical environment it is essential that anxieties and concerns as well as hopes and enthusiasm for new practices be openly shared and discussed.

Summary

The introduction of complementary therapies into current nursing practice carries with it many unique challenges and opportunities. It is, however, inextricably linked with the management of change. How an individual or group chooses to approach the process of change will influence the extent to which an innovative aspect of nursing care is accepted by the team as part of mainstream care.

Managing the introduction of complementary health care within orthodox nursing will, if strategically planned, take time. Many issues such as research, establishing safety and efficacy of therapies, policy development and standard setting, should form part of the process of change before therapies are practised in the clinical environment.

A knowledge of the process of change empowers and enables nurses proactively to manage and shape future nursing practice.

REFERENCES

Bennis W G, Benne K D, Chin R, Corey K E 1976 The planning of change. Holt Rinehart & Winston, London

Dobson C B, Hardy M, Heyes S, Humphreys A, Humphreys P 1988 Understanding psychology. Weidenfeld & Nicholson, London

Haffer A 1986 Facilitating change. Nursing Administration 16: 18–22

Keyzer D 1989 Meeting the challenge: strategies for implementing change. In: Wright S G (ed) Changing nursing practice. Edward Arnold, London

Lewin K 1953 Research studies in group decisions. Evanston, Row Peterson. Cited by: Brooten D A 1984 Managerial leadership in nursing. Lippincott, Philadelphia

Lippitt G 1970 Visualizing change: model building and the change process. New York Association. Cited by Brooten D A 1984 Managerial leadership in nursing. Lippincott, Philadelphia

Moss-Kanter R 1983 The change masters. Routledge, New York

Moss-Kanter R 1984 Managing the human side of change. AMACOM A Division of American Management Association. Reprinted from: Management Review April 1985 p 52–56

Seifert H, Clinebell H 1969 Personal growth and social change. Westminster, Philadelphia. Cited by: Brooten D A 1984 Managerial leadership in nursing. Lippincott, Philadelphia

Toffler A 1970 Future shock. Pan, London

Wright S G (ed) 1989 Changing nursing practice. Edward Arnold, London

4 Policy development

Maxine McVey

INTRODUCTION

To date there are few national guidelines determining the practice of complementary therapies. However, paragraph 39 of the UKCC Standards for the Administration of Medicines states that the practice of complementary therapies should be based upon sound principles, available knowledge and skill (UKCC 1992). A number of regional health authorities have developed policy statements and guidelines that stipulate forms and standards of practice (Bath 1991, West Berkshire 1992, St Bartholomew's 1993). This chapter examines a range of issues in policy development and the successful implementation of complementary therapies within clinical practice. Policy development currently falls within the remit of a working party established to address a range of issues associated with complementary therapies in the clinical setting. The establishment of a working party, its aims and subsequent policy development, is also discussed here.

A POLICY

A policy is a constitution, a course of action, a principle adapted or proposed by government party, business or an individual (Concise Oxford Dictionary 1990). Thus it is a set of guidelines sanctioned by those in authority, whether members of the trust board in a self-governed hospital or members of parliament. It states the intentions in a given situation, and guides good conduct in practical situations. Policy documents are commonly likened to codes of conduct or practices that define or establish principles and standards of practice.

RATIONALE FOR POLICY DEVELOPMENT IN COMPLEMENTARY THERAPIES

There are a number of reasons why a policy should be developed for the integration of complementary therapies into clinical practice. All qualified nurses are bound by the UKCC Code of Professional Conduct

(1992) and accountability is an integral part of this code. It is generally within the practical sphere that a nurse practitioner has to make judgements and be answerable for them. Policy documents usually state intentions in a given situation, with the aim of having the guidelines sanctioned by those in authority. As a rule, issues are addressed and where possible, solutions proposed. A policy further seeks to safeguard the safety of the patient and public.

In conjunction with the UKCC Scope of Professional Practice (1992), policy development in complementary therapies assists nurses towards identifying competent practice. In this respect, a policy promotes and classifies principles of practice directed at safeguarding the patient and the public. Additionally, policy development serves to reinforce the UKCC guidelines by highlighting issues associated with professional accountability within practice. A final consideration is the establishment of clear definitions and measurable criteria upon which clinical practice in this field can be evaluated. This latter aspect is important since it is the issue which will assist in determining efficiency of treatments.

SETTING UP A WORKING PARTY FOR COMPLEMENTARY THERAPIES

The team selected for policy development should be multidisciplinary. The members of the group are required to have a commitment to the aims of the working party, with each individual having a role to play to ensure the successful implementation of complementary therapies within the clinical setting. The team structure might be as follows:

- Membership/Trust manager — to provide information relating to cost and management issues

- Nurses who have an interest/qualification in complementary therapies — to have an understanding of the code of professional conduct; knowledge of the therapies — to evaluate practical issues related to their integration and implementation

- Health care professionals from different clinical areas — knowledge of different specialties to establish whether or not the policy is relevant to the nurses using it in a range of settings

- Multidisciplinary team, e.g. doctors, physiotherapists, pharmacists — to ensure collaboration between disciplines

- Links with other health policy initiatives and Department of Health developments towards research based practice

- If possible a person with experience of policy development — to facilitate policy development and assist in developing a framework defining the aims, objectives and issues relating to the formulation of a policy

When meetings involve more than ten people, individual participation becomes difficult. (Dobree 1991); initial teams of about five to seven members are recommended. Some members may only be required to attend a meeting when items relevant to their positions are discussed. Questions for initial consideration include:

- By whose authority is the group established?
- Is the group just to develop a policy?
- Is there a responsibility to establish how many nurses are practising complementary therapies in the hospital/region?
- Does the group have a role in encouraging and enabling therapies to be practised?
- Resource implications for facilitating committee meetings.

Organization of the team

In addition to team selection, the organization of the team should be addressed at initial meetings to set the framework for future decisions.

- Role of chairperson — the selection and the definition of the responsibilities as link person for communication within the group
- Secretarial support — the necessary skills to be able to fulfil the position, for example typing, recording minutes and administrative duties.
- Venue of meetings — if possible an identified place, away from distractions, e.g. clinical area
- Frequency of meetings — to maintain momentum and enable reflection and action between the meetings
- Timescale to produce a policy — objectives should be set, to be met before each meeting as well as an overall timescale for the development of a policy
- The remit of the group — additional roles identified; vice chair, remit of individuals.

The purpose of the group, its aims and objectives should be decided at the first meeting. This will guide the planning of the meetings and the activities of members and dictate when the project has been achieved.

Preliminary issues

In defining the remit and structure of the team, it will be necessary to identify the aims and objectives of the group. These may range from a defined focus on policy development to a broader remit whereby the group acts as a hospital or regional resource for matters relating to complementary therapies. The list below includes features attributable to professional practice and policy committees.

- Policy development for the use of complementary therapies
- Act as a resource for all nurses and health care professionals interested in complementary therapies
- Provide a forum for sharing and updating information in this field
- Clarify and establish organizational resources to support the development of complementary therapies.

Any policy development requires the establishment of baseline knowledge in order to define its remit. Methods of acquiring this include:

- Reviewing existing health authority policies on complementary therapies — identifying key issues to be addressed
- Conducting a literature search to appraise critically the substantive base upon which a therapy is established and therapeutic claims affirmed
- Organizing a survey to identify consumer demand for specific therapies within a hospital or region
- Establishing the current usage of specific therapies within nursing practice and identifying competent practitioners.

This list is a general guide and not exhaustive: the field is rapidly developing and therefore certain issues take on greater or lesser importance depending upon current social and political factors. It can be valuable to define clear terms of reference and in particular, links should be established with existing committees.

FACTORS TO CONSIDER WHEN FORMULATING A POLICY

Some areas commonly included in current policies addressing complementary therapies are as follows:

- Title of policy

- Identification of aim — overall goal
- Definition of terms used within the policy
- Identification of objectives — attainable goals that can be evaluated and measured
- Identification and evaluation of research studies on therapeutic efficacy and any treatment claims made
- Identification and critical evaluation of established training courses
- Identification of established organizations with recognized educational criteria in particular therapies
- Human resource issues — management
- Identification of educational criteria to determine competent practitioners within the hospital/health care region
- Definition of competency to practise
- Identification of existing registers of practitioners and criteria for inclusion on the register
- Evaluation of existing health policies in this field
- Establishment of links and possible inclusion of an experienced member of a previous policy development team on the proposed team
- Establishment of links with other organizations involved in development of complementary therapies within health care (e.g. the RCN Complementary Therapies in Nursing Forum)
- Identification of therapies/techniques to be included
- Definitions of and information about therapies
- Contraindications for use of certain therapies
- Professional bodies who may facilitate training and integration of a therapy in to the health care setting
- Development of a multidisciplinary team approach towards the use of therapies in the health care setting
- Evaluation of a therapy
- Financial considerations — cost-effectiveness of a therapy
- Ongoing research considerations
- Links between various regional policies
- Defining organizational responsibilities
- Identification of policy standards in line with national and European legislature

- Informed consent
- Insurance
- Documentation

Key issues

The key issues listed here are central to policy development. They are influenced by the clinical environment and the therapeutic modality to be used and some may be explored or defined in more detail according to the needs of specific clinical centres:

- Professional autonomy
- Accountability and responsibility
- Competency to practise
- Consent
- Consultation and collaboration
- General management issues
- Documentation
- Insurance

Accountability and responsibility

Accountability is inextricably linked with terms such as liability and responsibility. That many nurses interpret accountability and responsibility as being the same is understandable since the terms are frequently used interchangeably. Accountability originates from responsibility (Pearson & Vaughan 1990). Gardener (1992) states that accountability is dependent on knowledge, competence and experience. As knowledge and experience increase, competencies are more formally established. Some questions related to accountability in the use of complementary therapies and policy development are as follows:

- Are there specific issues to be addressed with specific therapies?
- What are the legal parameters of practice?
- Are those responsible for an area, accountable for that area?
- Are accountability and responsibility the same issue?
- Can a therapist be responsible and not accountable?
- Is accountability mandatory or a choice for the qualified nurse?
- What are the implications for accountability in relation to complementary therapies?

Lewis and Bate (1982) suggest accountability refers to 'formal obligation to disclose'. Thus, as a therapist you should be able to state:

- What it is you are trying to achieve — defining the goal in selecting and using a complementary therapy

- How you are trying to achieve it — selecting an action, the procedure involved in a therapy

- Why you are trying to achieve it — developing a knowledge base, being aware of and able critically to appraise the substantive research base underlying selected therapies

- The outcome of your actions — your evaluation, the development of an evaluation procedure for both the client and therapist.

As a nurse you must be able to give explanations for your actions and conduct, to answer as the one responsible (UKCC Scope of Professional Practice 1992). Binnie et al (1984) list three kinds of accountability:

- To the client or patient — a patient has the right to expect a service that maintains a high standard of care

- To the profession and the public throughout the UKCC — this is expressed in the code of professional conduct (UKCC 1992)

- To colleagues — most job descriptions contain a clause regarding the person(s) to whom nurses are accountable.

Accountability is often regarded as having to answer for an action when something goes wrong. It is actually more complex and is linked to evaluation, and how professional performance is monitored. Thus a critical appraisal of intended actions and the implications of those actions in their entirety should also be addressed. The implications of complementary therapies should be carefully thought through before practice and the nurse should evaluate whether she or he feels competent to practise (UKCC Scope of Professional Practice 1992).

Competency to practise

The Scope of Professional Practice (UKCC 1992) states that: 'the registered nurse, midwife or health visitor must be satisfied that each aspect of practice is directed to meeting the needs and serving the interests of the patient or client.' Being accountable is to some extent dependent upon having the authority and autonomy to act but this may not always occur. This relates to the nurse and manager agreeing to the use of the organization's resources. It is suggested that in complementary therapies authorization is directly linked with competency to practise in association with the development of a multidisciplinary team approach within the clinical setting and across the therapeutic specialism. It is necessary that each individual nurse recognizes personal competency skills and that these can be evaluated to ensure the client is safeguarded. Considerations may include:

- Safeguarding the patient/client
- Ensuring practice abides with the UKCC
- Recognizing limits to competency — not exceeding personal skills
- Defining criteria for a competent educational programme
- Recognizing contraindications to treatments
- Working within a multidisciplinary team — not countermanding medical instructions
- Promoting the safe and effective use of complementary therapies
- Demonstrating the ability to perform therapeutic techniques that can be evaluated and which meet established educational criteria.

Whilst many complementary therapies are frequently presented as an expansion of the nurse's role, certain therapies make definitive therapeutic and treatment claims. Some therapies claim diagnostic and treatment processes analogous to medicine, e.g. herbalism, acupuncture and to some extent aromatherapy. Where there is the potential for interaction with conventional medical treatment, collaborative multidisciplinary approaches to practice are needed. The General Medical Council guidelines for doctors, 'Professional Conduct and Discipline: Fitness to Practise' (GMC 1992), sets out conditions for the delegation of medical duties to nurses and others; paragraphs 42 and 43 of this document, state that doctors who delegate treatment or other procedures must ensure the person to whom they are delegated is competent to carry them out. It is, however, also appropriate to consider developing the nurse's role as a practitioner of complementary therapy independently of medically delegated duties.

Who is competent to practise? Answering this question may be fundamental to the aims of the group and affects the key issues formulating the criteria for the policy. Candidates include:

- Qualified staff with a recognized course
- A qualified nurse who has received instruction in a therapy and is under the supervision of the qualified staff with a recognized course

- A student or a care assistant
- A therapist who is not a nurse.

Competency through education. The patient/client is ethically protected by the UKCC and the nurse's professional responsibility. To help nurses considering a complementary therapy, guidelines have been formulated by the RCN, Department of Nursing Policy and Practice, Complementary Therapies in Nursing Special Interest Group (see Chapter 2 on Choosing a therapy). The significant aspects of training are:

- desirable course contents
- a period of supervision
- formal examination which enables a person to obtain insurance.

Consent

It is essential that policy documents address the issue of informed consent. Informed consent requires that the patient receives sufficient information to take a decision about the therapy and implies that the person giving the information has a sound knowledge base. If a nurse has insufficient information, clients should be referred to additional sources. Informed consent should be obtained before practice with the client receiving information about the therapy detailing benefits, contraindications and side effects. The main areas for policy consideration are as follows:

- Should consent be documented?
- What form should be used?
- What are the legal implications of developing a form?
- Can a formal consent form be completed by a therapist who is not a nurse?

Consultation and collaboration

When developing innovative clinical practice it is valuable to ensure multidisciplinary collaboration. This is linked to competency to practise and the safety of the clients. Questions for consideration include:

- How can this be achieved?
- Do specific therapies limit which patients/clients can be treated?
- Should the consultation be documented?
- What happens if a patient wishes to have a therapy and the medical practitioner is not in favour?

- What if the patient was using a therapy prior to being in the care of a medical practitioner?

The policy may not be able to answer all these questions; some issues will need to be resolved locally and not by policy.

General management issues

The effectiveness of the therapy needs to be considered from a managerial and human resources perspective. For example:

- Does the manager have a responsibility to ensure a nurse has credentials to practise?
- Can the manager justify the use of the organization's resources?
- Is a therapy cost-effective?
- Are there cost implications in relation to staff training?
- Is there a case for a clinical specialist — who may not be a nurse?
- What are the purchaser's/patient's views on complementary therapies?
- Is there financial means to conduct studies to determine cost efficiency and effectiveness of a therapy within health care and establish resources for a therapy?

Documentation

It is important to record the complementary therapy treatment in the patient's care plan and to evaluate its effectiveness. There is uncertainty about the true benefits of many therapies over and above the well-recognized 'placebo' response to therapy given by a committed carer. Therefore it is an integral aspect of professional nursing to document and evaluate each treatment. Nurses should be prepared to undertake more research into complementary therapies to enhance the credibility of their practice.

Insurance

It is advisable that a therapist has his/her own public liability insurance. A recognized course should enable the therapist to obtain this. The types of therapies that can be covered in the policy may be dictated by an indemnity insurance via a trade union or professional body. The RCN provides a list of therapies currently identified and covered by professional indemnity insurance. Additionally the health authority may wish to provide further cover. Check with the legal department of the health authority for guidelines.

Summary

The implementation of certain therapies within clinical practice is dependent on nurses taking the initiative and expanding their scope of practice. In incorporating therapies within nursing practice it is hoped that a more holistic approach to care can be achieved.

REFERENCES

Binnie A et al 1984 A systematic approach to nursing care. Open University Press, Milton Keynes

Complementary Therapies in Nursing Special Interest Group 1993 Choosing a complementary therapies course RCN, London

Concise Oxford Dictionary 1990, 8th edn. Clarendon Press, Oxford

Dobree L 1991 The meeting game. Nursing Standard 6: 45–47

Gardner J H 1992 Where the buck stops. Nursing 5: ?

GMC 1992 Professional Conduct and Discipline. Fitness to Practice, para. 42

Lewis F M, Bate M V 1982 Clarifying autonomy and accountability to nursing service — part 11. Journal of Nursing Administration

Pearson A, Vaughan B 1990 Nursing models for practice. Heinemann Nursing, Oxford, p 49

UKCC 1992 Code of Professional Conduct, 3rd edn. UKCC, London

UKCC 1992 Scope of Professional Practice. UKCC, London

UKCC 1992 Standards for the Administration of Medicines. UKCC, London

FURTHER READING – JOURNALS

Armstrong F, Waldren R 1991 A complementary strategy. Nursing Times 87: 34–35

Burke C, Kikora K 1992 Cancer — the dual approach. Nursing Times 88: 62–66

Crowther D 1991 Complementary therapy in practice. Nursing Standard 5: 25–27

Rankin-Box D 1991 Proceed with caution. Nursing Times 87: 34–36

Stevensen C 1992 Holistic power. Nursing Times 88: 68–70

UKCC 1992 Code of Professional Conduct, 3rd edn. UKCC, London

UKCC 1992 Standards For The Administration of Medicines. UKCC Section 39, London

UKCC 1992 The Scope of Professional Practice. UKCC, London

FURTHER READING – BOOKS

BMA 1993 Complementary medicine: new approaches to good practice. British Medical Association/Oxford University Press, Oxford

Buckman R, Sabbagh K 1993 Magic or medicine? An investigation into healing. Macmillan, London

Complementary therapy. London Nursing Times / Macmillan, 1993

Grant B 1993 Alternative health: A–Z of natural healthcare. Optima, London

Inglis B 1979 Natural medicine. Collins, London

Olsen K 1991 The encylopaedia of alternative health care. Piatkus, London

Rankin-Box D (ed) 1988 Complementary health therapies: a guide for nurses and the caring professions. Chapman and Hall, London

Stanway A (ed) 1987 The natural family doctor. Gaia, London

USEFUL ADDRESSES

British Holistic Medical Association
179 Gloucester Place
London NW1 6DX
Tel: 0171 262 5299

Centre for Complementary
Medicine (North West)
Director: Denise Rankin-Box
School of Health Studies
Stockport College of Further &
Higher Education
Wellington Road South
Stockport SK1 3UQ

RCN Complementary Therapies in
Nursing Forum
Chair: Denise Rankin-Box
Royal College of Nursing
20 Cavendish Square
London W1M OAB
Tel: 0171 409 333 X365

Research Council for
Complementary Medicine
60 Gt Ormond Street
London WC1N 3HR
Tel: 0171 833 8897

Institute of Complementary
Medicine
PO Box 194
London SE16 1QZ

HEALTH AUTHORITIES THAT HAVE PRODUCED POLICIES ON COMPLEMENTARY THERAPIES

Royal Berks & Battle Hospital Trust
Royal Berkshire Hospital
Craven Road
Reading RG1 5AN
West Berkshire Health Authority
1992

Royal United Hospital
Combe Park
Bath
Avon BA1 3NG
Bath District Health Authority 1989

St Mark's Hospital
City Road
London EC1V 2PS
St Bartholomew's NHS Group 1993
(Homerton, St Mark's, St Bartholomew's)

With thanks to the above Health Authorities who have given their permission to act as policy resources for people interested in developing policies in the field.

5 Research issues

Caroline Stevensen

INTRODUCTION

Audit and evaluation of developments in nursing practice are essential. The use of complementary therapies within clinical nursing is not new, but the variety of 'hands on' and other supportive techniques has recently increased. As with any other clinical approach, those working with complementary therapies need to demonstrate their benefit to patients as well as to justify the time, energy and expense invested in them and to identify any changes associated with their use. This requires research, a 'careful search', a 'systematic investigation towards increasing the sum of knowledge' (Schwarz et al 1988). This idea of research fills many nurses with fear and dread and the intention of this chapter is to demystify it and make it more 'user-friendly'.

THE AIMS OF RESEARCH

Clinical research aims to answer a clinical question rather than just prove a point about a complementary therapy. It is necessary to have an open mind and a genuine interest in the truth. To carry research through all its stages, from conception to publication, requires keen interest and commitment. From the outset, whether conducting the simplest pilot study or a complex, clinical trial, the researcher should have in mind what the research is trying to determine. The work could be designed to:

- Evaluate the overall effectiveness of a given therapy
- Determine the cost of a particular therapy in terms of time, equipment and human resources
- Assess the suitability of types of patients and different therapies offered
- Establish effectiveness so that funding for complementary therapies may be continued.

In research, quite simply, a question is asked and a method of answering it found. The research question should be simple and generally have a single objective. It should be possible to sum up the research idea in one sentence, e.g. does foot massage before bedtime produce a better quality and quantity of sleep in the elderly?

PRACTICAL ISSUES

Clinical research needs careful planning, as with any unfamiliar journey, to avoid getting lost along the way. A suitable checklist is as follows:

- Initially discuss the research idea with colleagues, being realistic about what can be achieved
- Assess the personnel available — are they sufficiently motivated?
- Is collaboration a possibility?
- Are advice and support available?
- What is the setting? Is there a suitable and definable patient group?
- How much time is available for research?
- Will the research be performed as a separate and additional task to existing clinical duties? If so, the research might be abandoned before completion due to the added strain — can some existing duties be delegated to other personnel?
- Are grants available for funding the research?

Funding bodies offering support for research either from a nursing perspective or in complementary medicine sometimes advertise in the nursing press; alternatively information can be obtained from libraries or the relevant organizations.

- Has the research been costed? Include, for example, equipment required, computers and software for data analysis, personnel to assist in research (e.g. statistician, psychologist, research expert, secretarial help), stationery, literature searches.
- Have all personnel who will be involved in or affected by the research been informed? This might require:
  - a teaching session where the research can be explained
  - making copies of the research proposal available
  - a checklist of people who need to be informed about the research

- consent from consultants whose patients will be involved in the trial
- Will informed consent be given and documented? A signed consent form is a legal requirement for studies involving active treatment. A clear information sheet about the research for patients and their supporters is needed. Careful and realistic consideration of all of these aspects will avoid difficulties later on which could result in failure of the research project. Equipment and expertise available locally should be sought out.

REVIEW OF THE COMPLEMENTARY THERAPIES LITERATURE

It is essential to read published studies relevant to the trial, both with regard to the therapy to be used and the condition treated. This can help to:

- see what has already been done in the research field and what conclusions have been reached by others
- understand different ways research can be performed in terms of methodology and assessment of outcome
- note the difficulties experienced by other researchers
- consider the structure of writing up research for publication.

Literature searches can be organized with the help of a good librarian. The Research Council in Complementary Medicine in London carries a database of complementary therapy research from which searches can be obtained (see useful addresses).

RESEARCH DESIGN

Choice of research design will primarily depend on the question being asked. It is affected by the ability to define a homogeneous group of patients in order to minimize extraneous variables. The patient subjects may have the same diagnosis and be grouped according to age and sex. Availability and access to the patients, dependent on factors such as length of stay or frequency of visits, will affect design. Inclusion and exclusion criteria should be defined to reduce variability. Simplicity in study design is recommended for any trial. There is little point spending time and energy collecting information that will never be analysed usefully.

Important aspects of research design

Controls are needed in any study to enable a group of similar patients to be compared with or without the therapy offered.

Randomization is performed so that the sample studied will be a valid representation of the whole population.

Independent assessment by personnel not involved in the performance of the therapy should always be used in the measurement of outcomes in order to reduce bias in the results.

Blinding of participants in the research to the treatment the patient receives is also used to reduce bias in the following three ways:

- 1, where the patient is unaware of which treatment was given (1: single blind)
- 2, where the performer of the research is unaware of the treatment given (1 and 2: double blind)
- 3, where the assessor of the trial outcomes is unaware of the treatment given (1 and 3: double blind; 1, 2 and 3: treble blind).

For example, massage is impossible to perform in a sham method that would not have some effect on the patient, but it is possible for the assessor not to know if the patient had massage or not.

Consistency and reliability

Testing research personnel for consistency of approach and standardization of the technique used is essential to reduce variability. Standardization of responses to the patient is also important in the research situation when the researcher is questioned. Reliability refers to the dependability of a test as reflected in the consistency of its scores upon repeated measurements of the same group. Validity refers to the ability of a test to measure what it is intended to measure. For example, a visual analogue scale used to measure pain relief before and after the administration of a complementary therapy could be considered reliable and valid if indeed pain was the variable chosen.

Choice of appropriate outcome measures

This can be problematic if examination of the holistic effects of a therapy is sought. Validated standardized measures of outcome are required. Measurements can be taken physiologically, psychologically or looking at effects on wellbeing and quality of life. The change of vital sign measurements can be transient in their effect from the use of massage (Stevensen 1994), whilst appropriate psychological measures are difficult to find. Have courage to adapt existing measures if they do not fit present requirements. Ease and simplicity is important from the patient's point of view. Visual analogue scales for measuring, clear questionnaires and the appropriate uses of open and closed questions can be used to obtain the information required.

Quantitative methods

The design aspects mentioned earlier are used so that comparisons between groups can be made statistically. To get a statistically significant result would suggest the definite advantage of one treatment compared with another. Quantitative methods are possible with physiological measurements where numerical data are presented, e.g. heart or respiratory rate, or existing psychological scales which have been quantified, e.g. the state anxiety inventory STAI form X-1 (Spielberger et al 1973). Statistical help should be sought before the trial starts to ensure an adequate sample size has been included for statistical analysis.

Qualitative methods

In some complementary therapies research, qualitative measures are more useful and appropriate as they examine how it is that people have come to knowledge and understanding (Powers & Knapp 1990); for example, describing how they feel after a certain therapy has been given or the benefits to nurses using complementary therapies in their practice. Rather than using statistics, measures of quality and accuracy are used. In practice this means that responses are classified into groups or units of meaning so that the researcher can better organize and make sense of the data (Burnard & Morrison 1990). The formation of categories of response also allows comparisons to be made between different groups of data. These groups may include feelings expressed, activities or comments about their treatment or condition or therapeutic setting (Burnard & Morrison 1990). In some instances, holistic complementary therapy research may lend itself more appropriately to the non-statistical format where the whole person can be taken into account as well as addressing the needs of the clinicians concerned (Aldridge 1993).

Writing the research proposal

This exercise helps to formulate the research in the mind of the researcher and sets a good foundation for the final research report. A proposal is also needed for submission to the ethical committee in order to obtain approval of the study.

The research proposal should contain the following:

- An introduction including reasons for undertaking the study
- A review of the literature
- The hypothesis to be investigated
- Consent form and patient information sheet
- Number of patients to be studied to meet statistical requirements
- The design and methodology
- Means of data collection for the study
- Methods of data analysis.

Ethical committee approval

This is required for clinically based research trials. The purpose of the ethical committee is to protect the patient from harmful practices and to ensure that the patient is not denied essential treatment as a result of the research process. When submitting a research proposal to the ethical committee, keep the information simple and free from unnecessary jargon and detail. Some committee members may not have heard of the complementary therapy to be used, whilst others may be experts.

Ethical considerations which should be addressed in research include the following:

- all issues related to the research, discussed with both the subjects and the association
- informed written consent
- right to privacy
- right to self-dignity
- assured confidentiality
- freedom from harm
- protection of patient's anonymity
- self-determination.

Data collection

Data collection should be organized such that it can be easily placed in a computer database or on a spreadsheet if quantitative. Qualitative data should be coded or grouped in some way. This will simplify the analysis of the information at the end of the data collection period and enable data to be stored in a meaningful way as the trial progresses.

Pilot studies

A pilot study should always be conducted and is particularly important for inexperienced researchers or new areas of research. It will enable the removal of any problems with the design and method of data collection that have not been previously anticipated.

Data analysis

Methods of data analysis should have been agreed before the formal part of the study starts. It must be clear what kinds of information are required and what will be measured and compared to what. Analysed data can be presented in various forms such as tables, graphs, bar charts, histograms and pie charts. Clarity to the reader is important; for example, several simpler charts are preferable to a complex one containing all the data.

Writing the research report

Writing the final report cannot be done until all other stages of the research process are completed. It is important to follow the standardized format and style that meet the requirements of the journal of choice for publication. The choice of journal will depend on the target audience for the research. Elements of the report generally include:

- Summary of the research and its major findings
- Introduction of the subject and literature review
- Methods, including
  - sample selection (inclusion and exclusion criteria)
  - study design
  - outcome measures
- Results
- Discussion, including
  - limitations of the study
  - how the research contributes to the wider body of knowledge in the field
  - further research that could be performed.

Summary

Research in complementary therapies within nursing is an important and exciting development. Despite this being a relatively new area of research, standard techniques can be applied. Some difficulties could be encountered over the appropriate choice of outcome measures which reflect the holistic nature of the therapy given and the maintenance of patient individuality as well as the potential benefits offered. Reference to research in this field already performed by nurses and other health care professionals will provide support to those embarking on trials. Good research in complementary therapies will answer questions as to their effectiveness for use in and out of the orthodox health care setting.

REFERENCES

Aldridge D 1993 Research strategies in a hospital setting: the development of appropriate methods. In: Lewith G T, Aldridge D (eds) Clinical research methodology for complementary therapies. Hodder & Stoughton, London

Burnard P, Morrison P 1990 Nursing research in action. Macmillan Education Basingstoke, Hampshire

Powers B A, Knapp T R 1990 A dictionary of nursing theory and research. Sage, CA, USA

Schwarz C et al (eds) 1988 Chambers English dictionary. Chambers, Cambridge

Spielberger C D, Gorsuch R L, Lushene R 1973 Self evaluation questionnaire STAI Form X-1. Consulting Psychologists Press, CA, USA

Stevensen C J 1994 The psychophysiological effects of aromatherapy massage on the post cardiac surgery patient. Complementary Therapies in Medicine 2: 27–35

FURTHER READING – JOURNALS

Aldridge D 1989 A guide to preparing a research application. Complementary Medical Research 3: 31–37

Anthony H M 1989 Clinical research: questions to ask and the benefits of asking them. Complementary Medical Research 3: 3–5

James I 1989 Tactics and practicalities. Complementary Medical Research 3: 7–10

Mills S 1991 Herbal medicines: research strategies. Complementary Medical Research 5: 29–35

Pocock S 1989 Error and bias in single-group and controlled data. Complementary Medical Research 3: 11–13

FURTHER READING – BOOKS

Brink P J, Wood M J 1989 Advanced design in nursing research. Sage, CA, USA

Cormack D F S (ed) 1991 The research process in nursing, 2nd edn. Blackwell Scientific, Oxford

Grady K E, Wallston B S 1988 Research in health care settings. Sage, CA, USA

Herbert M 1990 Planning a research project: a guide for practitioners and trainers in the helping professions. Castle Education, London

Hockey L 1985 Nursing research: mistakes and misconceptions. Churchill Livingstone, Edinburgh

McNeil P 1985 Research methods. Tavistock, London

Reid N G, Boore J R P 1987 Research methods and statistics in health care. Edward Arnold, London

Robson C 1993 Real world research: a resource for social scientists and practitioner researchers. Blackwell, Oxford

USEFUL ADDRESS

Research Council for
Complementary Medicine
60 Great Ormond Street
London WC1N 3HR
Tel: 0171 833 8897

SECTION 2

Therapies

6 Acupuncture

Stephanie Downey

Acupuncture — *a Chinese medical system which aims to diagnose illness and promote health by stimulating the body's self-healing powers.*

In the last three decades there has been a significant increase in the acceptance of acupuncture within western medical practice. Recognized by the British Medical Association (BMA) as a 'discrete clinical discipline' (BMA 1993), acupuncture now faces the challenge of biomedical integration and the need to adapt to western needs whilst still retaining the integrity of its oriental tradition.

Acupuncture involves the insertion of fine needles into specific points on the body. The word derives from the Latin *acus* (needle) and *punctura* (puncture). Behind this apparently simple technique, lies a rich and complex theoretical system rooted in Confucian and Taoist philosophy and developed and refined over 2000 years through extensive observation and clinical evaluation.

Central to the theory behind acupuncture is the concept of the body as a self-healing, self-rectifying, dynamic whole, a network of interrelating and interacting energies (Firebrace & Hill 1988). The even distribution and flow of these energies maintains health, and through the insertion of needles acupuncture helps the body to correct itself by realigning or redirecting the energy. A related technique, moxibustion, involves the application of heat from the burning of the herb mugwort (*Artemisia vulgaris*) at the acupuncture points. This has a warming, moving and strengthening effect on the body.

Acupuncture is but one aspect of traditional Chinese medicine that includes herbs, diet, massage and exercise. All of these techniques developed on the basis of principles (Bejing College of Traditional Medicine et al 1980) which see the body as inseparable from its environment, a microcosm of the universe and permeated with the same energy. In the human body this energy, or Qi, is dispersed through 12 main channels (meridians) all following fixed pathways to connect the different levels from the internal organs to the skin. Illness occurs primarily when there is excess, deficiency or obstruction of the energy within the organs or meridian pathways. For example, symptoms such as arthritic pain in the hips, intercostal neuralgia or migraine headaches would suggest an imbalance in the Gall Bladder, whose meridian traverses the lateral sides of the body from the foot to the temples. Likewise, pain and stiffness in the arm of someone with repetitive strain injury may be due to blocked Qi in the Large Intestine meridian which runs from the index finger to the elbow. Similarly, a deficiency of energy in the Lungs can manifest as dyspnoea, asthma or a tendency to catch colds. The aim of acupuncture in each case is to regulate and correct imbalances of Qi and so assist the body's own recuperative powers.

The dynamic balance of energy central to acupuncture can be expressed by the concepts of Yin and Yang. In Chinese medicine, Yin/Yang describe patterns of disharmony and are relative rather than absolute terms. Yang is characterized by heat, movement, activity and excess, whereas Yin relates more to cold, sluggishness, inactivity and deficiency. A balance of each kind of energy is necessary for health.

A further refinement of Yin/Yang is the Five Elements or Phases. This is a system of correspondences which include organs/meridians, emotions, seasons and climates, linked to the elements of Fire, Earth, Metal, Water and Wood in a dynamic cycle of creation and control. For example:

- Fire: Heart/Small Intestine, joy, summer, heat
- Earth: Spleen/Stomach, obsession, late summer/between seasons, dampness
- Metal: Lungs/Large Intestine, sadness/grief, autumn, dryness
- Water: Kidney/Bladder, fear/fright, winter, cold
- Wood: Liver/Gall Bladder, anger, spring, wind.

The inter-relating energies are governed by this relationship, so that an imbalance in one area will lead to a breakdown of the cycle causing disharmony within other elements and manifesting as physical or emotional disorders within the associated organ/meridian.

The existence of Qi and channels cannot be explained, as yet, within the parameters of western science. Acupuncture has been shown to have an effect on biochemical, neurological and hormonal systems. However, none of these paradigms is adequate to account for the permanent changes acupuncture can mobilize in some aspects of physiological behaviour; for example, in chronic headaches (Bensoussan 1991).

The World Health Organization (Bannerman 1979) recognizes the efficacy of acupuncture in the treatment of over 40 diseases. While its use in the west is often limited to chronic conditions, the integration of traditional and modern medicine in China has shown acupuncture to be remarkably successful in the treatment of more serious and acute diseases such as appendicitis, cholecystitis, renal colic and the sequelae of cerebrovascular accident (Deadman 1982). For acupuncture to find its true place within the medical services it is important that it is used in the hospital system alongside biomedicine.

To ensure its future as a complete medical system, acupuncture faces three major issues: training, regulatory procedures and research. The Council for Acupuncture provides a forum for the five professional bodies who keep registers of their members, and has established the British Acupuncture Accreditation Board (BAAB). This seeks to accredit colleges on the basis of compliance with established minimum standards of training (Shifrin 1993, Uddin 1993).

While research into acupuncture is prolific in China and has increased in the west (Bensoussan 1991), this has largely been modelled on the empirical methods that dominate the natural sciences. The extent to which Chinese medicine can be understood or evaluated within the current framework of conventional western science requires urgent attention (Scheid 1993).

HISTORICAL BACKGROUND

The origin of acupuncture in China is not clear. Although excavations have revealed the existence of stone needles dating back to 3000 BC, the earliest document, the *Huangdi NeiJing*, was probably written between 300 and 100 BC (Maciocia 1982). Translated as the *Yellow Emperor's Classic of Internal Medicine*, this work lays down the theoretical foundations of Chinese medicine and is still frequently cited in modern acupuncture textbooks. In the second century BC acupuncture was adopted as the dominant therapeutic technique (Unschuld 1985) and later centuries saw the development of the main acupuncture theories relating to meridian systems, Yin/Yang, the Five Elements, the nature and types of Qi, the functions of the organs and their pathology. The popularity and acceptance of different schools of thought regarding Chinese medical theories varied throughout Chinese history in response to shifts in religious behaviour and sociopolitical ideologies.

After the Opium War in 1840, biomedicine as part of western science and technology came to China and traditional medicine was marginalized. Since the formation of the People's Republic in 1949, Chinese medicine has been actively encouraged and systematized.

Knowledge of acupuncture in Europe was generally derived from reports by travelling doctors and treatises by Jesuit missionaries working in China in the seventeenth century (Hsu 1989). Gaining popularity initially in France and Germany, acupuncture spread to Britain and has become increasingly widespread since the 1960s.

TREATMENT

Although acupuncture has gained prominence in the west as a method of pain relief, its efficacy extends to disorders of the respiratory, digestive and nervous systems as well as emotional and psychological problems.

The diagnostic process, whereby signs and symptoms are pieced together and synthesized until a picture of the whole person appears, is integral to the application of acupuncture. An initial consultation will address the current problem as well as eliciting information about emotional state, exposure to adverse climatic conditions, trauma, accidents, hereditary factors, diet and social factors, all of which are seen to interact to disrupt the flow of Qi. Diagnosis will also be based on the person's appearance, facial colour and posture. Finally, the pulse will be palpated and the tongue observed to provide additional information about the energetic balance and state of Qi within the organs and meridians.

The diagnosis is made according to the theoretical framework of traditional Chinese medicine. Most important is the recognition of the uniqueness of each individual's condition. Two people may present with the diagnostic label of arthritis, yet one may experience a fixed biting pain aggravated by cold and have a pale tongue and slow pulse, while the other may have migratory pain, red hot swollen joints, red tongue and a rapid pulse. The diagnosis and treatment will be tailored to the individual. As well as inserting fine needles into specific points on the body, moxibustion may be applied, and each subsequent treatment will vary in the points used, according to the particular recovery pattern. The therapeutic basis in traditional terms of acupuncture stimulation is that by restoring the flow of Qi within the channels, the 'vital energy' of the organism is regulated (reinforced or reduced) and thus restores balance, improves body resistance and helps to eliminate pathogenic factors (Hillier & Jewell 1983).

Therapeutic potential in nursing

There are many opportunities for nurses to practise acupuncture, although only a full training in traditional Chinese medicine will prevent acupuncture becoming just another biomedical technique. The nursing role may also need to be re-examined as well as the extent to which holistic care can be provided within the constraints of traditional nursing models (Burke 1993).

Potential areas for acupuncture in nursing include:

- Pain management — post-operatively, in out-patient clinics, accident and emergency departments
- Sports medicine — in conjunction with physiotherapy
- Obstetrics — pain relief, induction of labour, turning the fetus in breech presentation
- Oncology — control of emesis after chemotherapy
- Occupational health
- Mental health — emotional distress
- Drug rehabilitation centres — control of withdrawal symptoms
- Treatment of HIV/AIDS as part of a multidisciplinary team.

Contraindications for use

Certain behaviour is thought to affect the state of Qi and may counteract the effect of acupuncture or occasionally result in dizziness. In general the following should be avoided immediately before and directly after treatment (Luwen 1990):

- alcohol
- excessive fatigue and hunger
- large meals
- sexual activity
- hot baths
- extreme emotional states.

In pregnancy there are no absolute contraindications, but some restrictions (Zharkin 1990) as follows:

- Moxibustion is not recommended, apart from certain specific points
- Certain points should not be needled during the first and second trimesters, or points below the umbilicus on the anterior abdominal wall.

Summary

Acupuncture has been shown to be effective in the treatment of a wide range of diseases. It may be used in a number of health care settings such as pain clinics, paediatrics and midwifery. However, care should be taken to ensure practitioners are well qualified, and where possible, acupuncture should be used to treat the whole person rather than for symptomatic relief.

REFERENCES

Bannerman R H 1979 Acupuncture: the WHO view. World Health (December) p 24–29

Bejing College of Traditional Chinese Medicine et al 1980 Essentials of Chinese acupuncture. Foreign Language Press, Bejing

Bensoussan A 1991 The vital meridian. Churchill Livingstone, Melbourne

BMA 1993 Complementary medicine. Oxford University Press, Oxford

Burke C 1993 Cancer nursing: complementary/conventional approaches combine. Complementary Therapies in Medicine 1: 158–163

Deadman P 1982 Report on the first international course for further students in acupuncture and moxibustion. Journal of Chinese Medicine 9: 1–5

Firebrace P, Hill S 1988 New ways to health — a guide to acupuncture. Hamlyn, London

Hillier S M, Jewell J A 1983 Health care and traditional medicine in China, 1800–1982. Routledge & Kegan Paul, London p 251

Hsu E 1989 Outline of the history of acupuncture in Europe. Journal of Chinese Medicine 29: 28–32

Luwen G 1990 Understanding the theory of acupuncture contraindications according to the NeiJing. Journal of Chinese Medicine 34: 31–32

Maciocia G 1982 History of acupuncture. Journal of Chinese Medicine 9: 9–15

Scheid V 1993 Orientalism revisited. European Journal of Oriental Medicine 1: 22–31

Shifrin K 1993 Setting standards for acupuncture training — a model for complementary medicine. Complementary Therapies in Medicine 1: 91–95

Uddin J 1993 The BMA report. European Journal of Oriental Medicine 1: 50–51

Unshuld P 1985 Medicine in China: a history of ideas. University of California Press, Berkeley

Zharkin N 1990 Acupuncture in obstetrics. Journal of Chinese Medicine 33: 10–13

FURTHER READING – JOURNALS

Christensen P A 1989 Electro-acupuncture and post-operative pain. British Journal of Anaesthesia 62: 258–262

Huang X 1994 The treatment of 114 cases of chemotherapeutic leucopenia by cone moxibustion. Journal of Chinese Medicine 44: 22–23

Knapman J 1993 Controlling emesis after chemotherapy. Nursing Standard 7: 38–39

Richardson P H, Vincent C A 1986 Acupuncture for the treatment of pain: a review of evaluative research. Pain 24: 15–40

Rossano N A 1992 Crack-cocaine abuse: acupuncture as an effective adjunct to therapy in current treatment programs. International Journal of Clinical Acupuncture 3: 333–338

Taylor B 1990 Acupuncture — a balancing act. Openmind 43: 12–14

Trevelyan J, Booth B 1994 Complementary medicine for nurses, midwives and health visitors. Macmillan Press, Houndmills, Basingstoke

Tsuei J J et al 1974 Induction of labour by acupuncture and electrical stimulation. Obstetrics and Gynaecology 43: 337–342

Woodier N C, Price P 1984 Acupuncture and its role in occupational health. Occupational Health (September) 406–416

FURTHER READING – BOOKS

Auteroche B et al 1992 Acupuncture and moxibustion: a guide to clinical practice. Churchill Livingstone, Edinburgh

Bensoussan A 1991 The vital meridian: a modern exploration of acupuncture. Churchill Livingstone, Melbourne

Kaptchuk T 1983 The web that has no weaver. Congdon & Weed, New York

Maciocia G 1989 The foundations of Chinese medicine. Churchill Livingstone, Edinburgh

Shanghai College of Traditional Medicine 1981 Acupuncture: a comprehensive text. Eastland Press, Chicago

USEFUL ADDRESSES

British College of Acupuncture
8 Hunter Street
London WC1N 1BN

College of Integrated Chinese
Medicine
40 College Road
Reading RG6 1QB
Tel: 01734 263366

Council for Acupuncture
179 Gloucester Place
London NW1 6DX
Tel: 0171 724 5756

London School of Acupuncture and
Traditional Chinese Medicine
36/37 Featherstone Street
London EC1Y 8QX

Northern College of Acupuncture
124 Acomb Road
York YO2 0EY
Tel: 01904 785120

British Medical Acupuncture
Society (BMAS)
Newton House
Newton Lane
Whitley
Warrington
Cheshire
WA4 4 JA

7 Aromatherapy

Caroline Stevensen

Aromatherapy — *a form of treatment using essential oils extracted from plants for therapeutic effect.*

'Aroma' literally means a spicy fragrance (Chambers 1988) and a popular misconception about aromatherapy is that it is simply the inhalation of pleasant perfumes with little therapeutic value. Whilst inhalation is an important part of aromatherapy, and indeed the oils can be used in this way or as room perfumers, the oils can also be absorbed through the skin when added to vegetable oil for massage (Balacs 1992), dropped in a bath or, as in France, taken orally if prescribed by trained doctors.

There are many therapeutic essential oils. They can be used to relax or invigorate the individual, and also for specific conditions; for example:

- lavender (*Lavandula latifolia*) for first-aid of burns (Franchomme & Penoel 1990)
- neroli (*Citrus aurantium* subspecies *aurantium*) for anxiety (Franchomme & Penoel 1990, Stevensen 1994)
- tea tree (*Muleleuca alternifolia*) for its antibacterial and antifungal action (Franchomme & Penoel 1990).

How essential oils work is not entirely understood despite scientific research, but this does not necessarily detract from their therapeutic value (Valnet 1990). It is thought that chemical properties of the essential oils, when absorbed in the body, have certain therapeutic benefits. Some therapists believe that the essential oil is the 'soul' of the plant, having both powerful and subtle properties that uplift the spirit as well as assisting with more fundamental health problems of body and mind.

HISTORICAL BACKGROUND

The use of plant extracts for health and wellbeing has been documented since records began. It is estimated that as far back as 40 000 years, Australian aborigines developed a knowledge of native plants for medicinal purposes which is still in use today. An example is the valuable antibacterial and antifungal properties of the Australian tea tree (*Maleleuca alternifolia*), the essential oil of which is used in modern aromatherapy (Blackwell 1991, Franchomme & Penoel 1990). Many ancient civilizations have used aromatic products. In 4500 BC, Kiwant Ti, a Chinese emperor, recorded therapeutic properties of plants that match those ascribed to them today (Arcier 1990). The ancient Egyptians used herbal oils to embalm bodies in preparation for the next life. Priests of that period were also doctors and used herbs and oils for the treatment of the sick as well as for beauty (Tisserand 1990). In the Bible, many references are made to plant oils. Moses was instructed to make a holy anointing oil from myrrh, calamus, cinnamon, cassia and olive oil (Exodus: chapter 30, verses 22–26). Frankincense and myrrh were reported to have been brought to the Christ child at his birth (Gospel according to St Matthew: chapter 2, verse 11). Plant oils continued to be used down the ages by the Hebrews, Greeks and Romans. Hippocrates, the father of modern medicine, several hundred years BC, commended a daily scented bath and massage for good health.

The first distillation of essential oils is formally attributed to the Arab scholar, Avicenna, in the tenth century AD. However, archeological evidence from the Indus Valley civilization suggests that this technique was known 5000 years earlier (Williams 1989). The use of plant oils continued throughout the Middle Ages up to modern times. Therapeutic use of essential oils this century is attributed to the French chemist R M Gattefosse (Franchomme & Penoel 1990). After severely burning his hand in a laboratory accident, he plunged it into a vat of lavender oil to find that the wound healed remarkably quickly and with no scarring. He coined the term 'aromatherapie' and his book of the same name describing his discoveries and experiences was published in 1931. Further research was carried out by Dr Jean Valnet in the 1960s, and the publication of his book *The practice of aromatherapy* (Valnet 1990) began a new wave of interest in the subject. The use of aromatherapy in nursing has been a developing trend through the 1980s. The increasing amount of nursing research on the clinical effectiveness of aromatherapy is encouraging (Dunn 1992, Stevensen 1994), although more clinical trials are needed.

TREATMENT

The properties of essential oils

Each essential oil is composed of chemical components thought to give it its individual therapeutic properties (Franchomme & Penoel 1990):

- Alcohols (C10): nervous system tonics, anti-infectious+++, immunostimulants
- Alcohols (C15–C20): oestrogen-like action
- Aldehydes: sedatives, anti-infectious, litholytic
- Aromatic aldehydes: anti-infectious+++, immunostimulants
- Coumarins and lactones: sedative, calming and anticoagulant
- Esters: relaxants, antispasmodics
- Ketones: mucolytic, lipolytic and cicatrizing
- Oxides: expectorants, antiparasitic
- Phenols: balance the autonomic nervous system, antispasmodics, anti-infectious+++, immunostimulants
- Terpenes (C10): cortisone-like action
- Terpenes (C15): antihistamine, antiallergic.

Some of these chemicals, such as ketones and phenols, can be toxic in large quantities or in patients with certain conditions, for example pregnancy or epilepsy. Understanding the chemical components of each oil is a necessary part of professional aromatherapy. For example, rosemary (*Rosmarinus officinalis*) essential oil has differing levels of toxicity depending on its chemotype or chemical subgrouping; the verbenone form has a higher risk of ketone toxicity than the borneone form.

The quality and chemical contents of essential oils are determined by their growing conditions, altitude and weather patterns, as well as the method of extraction. Essential oils are extracted principally by distillation, but other methods such as maceration, expression and solvent extraction are used depending on the source of the oil. Essential oils should be grown organically without chemical fertilizers and distilled without the addition of any other chemicals. Essential oils can be adulterated or extended with synthetic chemicals to increase productivity or to stabilize the perfume (as is required in the cosmetic industry). This will reduce or remove therapeutic effect and increase levels of toxicity in some oils. In addition, if the process of distillation is cut short, some therapeutic effects may be lost as more time is needed to extract certain chemical components. For example, if distillation is incomplete some of the sedating and calming effects of lactones and coumarins contained in lavender oil may be lost.

Information about the source of essential oils and standard of production should be available from any company selling them for therapeutic purposes. Poorly produced and identified oils could place patients at risk of skin reactions or more serious toxic reactions. Each essential oil has internationally accepted levels for its chemical components, which can be analysed by liquid gas chromatography (Franchomme & Penoel 1990, Williams 1989). It should be possible to obtain all this information from a reliable supplier.

Storage of essential oils

Essential oils must be stored in dark-coloured glass bottles as their constituents are affected by light. Plastic containers can adversely affect oils. As essential oils are volatile and evaporate easily, bottles should be firmly sealed and stored away from heat. Undiluted oils will keep for several years, whilst diluted oils may keep up to 12 months if stored correctly.

Administration of essential oils

There are several methods by which aromatherapy can be administered in a nursing context:

- massage: diluted with a vegetable oil
- inhalation: in a bowl of hot water, as a nebulizer, on a tissue, via a room fragrancer
- in a bath: 3–6 drops, soaking for at least 10 minutes.

Massage

This is a common form of administration since the beneficial effects of touch in combination with appropriate essential oils provide a supportive form of treatment for a variety of problems. Massage can be given to the whole body or to parts, as time permits. Professional training in massage and aromatherapy ensures the correct choice of essential oils and their dilutions in vegetable carrier oils, and appropriate massage techniques. In massage, oils absorbed into the bloodstream via the skin have a systemic effect (Balacs 1992).

Inhalation

Inhalation of oils affects the body, as the olfactory nerve fibres are directly linked with the limbic system of the brain, the emotional centre (Mosby 1983). Odours affects mood and can prompt memory of past events, happy or sad, so choice of oils is important. Inhalation also takes place when the oils are given via other routes. The essential oils of eucalyptus (*Eucalyptus radiata* ssp. *radiata*) or benzoin (*Styrax benzoe*) have been used by nurses for respiratory inhalations for many years. A drop of true lavender (*Lavandula angustifolia* ssp. *angustifolia*) on a tissue has been reported by nurses to assist sleep in the elderly, confirming some laboratory experiments (Guillemain et al 1989).

Therapeutic potential in nursing

Essential oils can be used for a wide range of conditions including:

- stress, anxiety and depression
- insomnia and restlessness
- acute asthma attacks and other respiratory conditions
- common colds and influenza
- digestive disorders, constipation
- muscular and neuralgic pain
- arthritis
- menstrual irregularities, thrush
- headaches and migraine
- burns, eczema, psoriasis and a variety of other skin conditions
- wound and scar healing
- during pregnancy and labour (see contraindications).

Contraindications for use

- If essential oils are administered with massage, then the contraindications for massage apply
- Essential oils must always be diluted before applying to the skin; the dilution will depend on the particular essential oil used and the age, size and condition of the patient
- Sensitive patients or those with allergies should be treated with caution; a simple patch test of the proposed blend of oils should be applied, if in doubt, before proceeding with full massage

- Oils for inhalation via fragrancers should be selected for individual patients rather than a whole ward
- Toxicity and contraindications for each oil must be well understood
- Keep essential oils away from eyes and mucous membranes
- In pregnancy, many oils are contraindicated due to toxic risk to mother and fetus or risk of spontaneous abortion. These include: aniseed, armoise (mugwort), arnica, basil, camomile (avoid in first trimester as it can induce menstruation), camphor, cedar, cinnamon, clary sage, clove, cypress, fennel, hyssop, jasmine, juniper, lavender (*Lavandula stoechas* not at any time; *L. angustifolia* ssp. *angustifolia* not during the first trimester), marjoram, myrrh, niaouli, origanum, pennyroyal, peppermint, sage, savory, rose, rosemary, ravensara, thuja, thyme and wintergreen. Fennel can be used as a tea for morning sickness, but do not use the essential oil (Davis 1988, Franchomme & Penoel 1990)
- Many of the oils just listed are toxic and not recommended for general use; oils that can be toxic for babies and young children include aniseed, hyssop, some eucalyptus, peppermint, fennel, myrrh, niaouli, camphor, ravensara, sage, thuja
- Do not use oils that elicit a negative psychological response from the patient (ask them)
- Due to the strong association that smell can have with memory, special care should be taken with patients undergoing chemotherapy or those feeling very unwell or sensitive; the smell of the same oil in a subsequent context could induce nausea, vomiting or negative emotions
- Aromatherapy is not for dabblers — undergo professional training before treating patients.

Summary

The use of aromatherapy in nursing practice has great potential. The benefits of essential oils have been known for centuries. Good practice requires sound knowledge of the chemical properties of essential oils and their therapeutic indications and contra-indications. In addition, practical experience is needed to apply aromatherapy appropriately in nursing. Further nursing research on aromatherapy in the clinical setting will improve understanding of this useful form of complementary therapy.

REFERENCES

Arcier M 1990 Aromatherapy. Hamlyn, London

Balacs T 1992 Dermal crossing. International Journal of Aromatherapy 4: 23–25

Blackwell A L 1991 Tea tree oil and anaerobic (bacterial) vaginosis (Letter). Lancet 337, 300

Chambers 1988 Chambers English Dictionary. Chambers, Cambridge

Davis P 1988 Aromatherapy: A–Z. CW Daniels, Saffron Walden, UK

Dunn C 1992 A report on a randomised controlled trial to evaluate the use of massage and aromatherapy in an intensive care unit. Battle Hospital, Reading, unpublished

Franchomme P, Penoel D 1990 L'aromatherapie exactement. Roger Jallois, Limoges

Guillemain J, Rousseau A, Delaveau P 1989 Neurodepressive effects of the essential oil of *Lavandula angustifolia* Mill. (French) Annales Pharmaceutiques Francaises 47: 337–343

Mosby C V 1983 Mosby's medical and nursing dictionary. CV Mosby, St Louis, USA

Stevensen C J 1994 The psychophysiological effects of aromatherapy following cardiac surgery. Complementary Therapies in Medicine 2: 27–35

Tisserand R 1980 The art of aromatherapy. CW Daniels, Saffron Walden, UK

Valnet J 1990 The practice of aromatherapy. CW Daniels, Saffron Walden, UK

Williams D 1989 Lecture notes on essential oils. Eve Taylor, London

FURTHER READING – JOURNALS

Buckle J 1993 Does it matter which lavender oil is used? Nursing Times 89: 32–35

Dale A, Cornwall S 1994 The role of lavender oil in relieving perineal discomfort following childbirth: a blind randomised clinical trial. Journal of Advanced Nursing 19: 89–96

van Toller S, Dodd G H 1983 The biology and psychology of perfumery. Perfumer Flavorist 8: 1–14

Torri S, Fukada H, Kanemoto H et al 1988 Contingent negative variation and the psychological effects of odour. In: van Toller S, Dodd G H (eds) Perfumery: the psychology and biology of fragrance. Chapman and Hall, London

FURTHER READING – BOOKS

Day K, White J 1992 Aromatherapy for scentual awareness. Nacson & Sons, NSW, Australia

Martin G 1989 Alternative health: aromatherapy. Optima, London

Tisserand M 1990 Aromatherapy for women. Thorsens, Wellingborough

Worwood V 1990 The fragrant pharmacy. Macmillan, London

USEFUL ADDRESSES

Aromatherapy Organisations
Council (AOC)
3 Laymers Close
Bray Carook
Market Harborough LE16 8LL
Tel: 01455 615 466

International Federation of
Aromatherapists (IFA)
Department of Continuing
Education
Royal Masonic Hospital
Ravenscourt Park
London W6 0TN
Tel: 0181 846 8066

International Society for
Professional Aromatherapists
(ISPA)
41 Leicester Road
Hinckley
Leicestershire LE10 1LW
Tel: 01455 637 987

Register of Qualified
Aromatherapists
54a Gloucester Avenue
London NW1 8JD

8 Autogenic training

Dorothy Crowther

Autogenic training — a psychophysiologic form of psychotherapy, which the patient carries out himself by using passive concentration upon certain combinations of psychophysiologically adapted verbal stimuli. Luthe (1963)

Autogenic training is not simply another relaxation method. The patient becomes a passive observer in the autogenic state (altered state of consciousness) while the brain's self-regulatory mechanism functions normally, thus allowing homoeostasis (rebalancing) to take place. Over 80 physiological changes have been measured during autogenic practice, demonstrating that a normalizing process takes place (Bafatt 1993).

The technique is easy to learn as it involves simple mental exercises that can be carried out anywhere, in an airport lounge, travelling by train, at work, and so on. Unlike many other therapies, autogenic training is not reliant upon a therapist; it is a self-empowering tool that once learned can be used whenever required. An adaptable technique, it is ideal for nurses to teach to patients, provided they have the contact time.

HISTORICAL BACKGROUND

Autogenic training was developed in Germany in the 1920s by the neuropsychiatrist Dr Johannes Schultz, after observing the work of Professor Oscar Vogt, an eminent researcher on psychophysiological changes of different states of conscious control (known as prophylactic rest periods). Shultz recognized the benefit of prophylactic rest periods to psychiatric patients and this led him to develop the standard exercises that provide the framework of autogenic training.

The original method was extended when Shultz met Dr Wolfgang Luthe in 1940. Research on specific problems in psychiatric patients, led Luthe to design techniques complementary to the standard exercises of autogenic training (Luthe & Schulz 1969). Dr Luthe left Germany for Canada where he continued work on autogenic training. In 1960, he introduced the concept of autogenic neutralization for those who required more than the standard exercises. This involved a consistently longer period in the autogenic state and was, according to Coleman (1988), intended to help psychiatric patients reach a 'curative' state of mental equilibrium. The extent of Luthe's work is seen in six volumes on autogenic therapy and its applications (see Further Reading — Books). Luthe's dedication to autogenic training led him to establish research centres in Canada and Japan and there are estimated to be over 3000 scientific papers on autogenic training. (Crocker & Grozelle 1991, Kaufman et al 1988).

In 1979, Dr Carruthers and his wife Vera Diamond, a psychotherapist, went to Canada to learn autogenic training. They recognized the benefits of this therapy for those at risk from stress-related illness and, in 1980, introduced autogenic training to Britain. In 1984, the British Association of Autogenic Training and Therapy (BAFATT) was set up for the regulation of training, maintaining professional standards and promoting research.

TREATMENT

Since autogenic training can have a profound effect on an individual, careful assessment and screening must take place. Usually, the patient is interviewed by the trainer to find out why they wished to learn autogenic training, since the work requires full cooperation. A full medical history covering physical, psychological, social and spiritual wellbeing is taken. A letter and a short medical questionnaire are also given to the patient to take to their General Practitioner; this informs the doctor that their patient wishes to undertake autogenic training and the returned questionnaire gives the trainer relevant medical information (with the patient's permission).

This method can be taught in small groups of four to six people or individually, depending upon the patient's preference; both methods are effective and streamlined according to individual need. Autogenic training requires eight weekly sessions with two follow-up sessions. Each session lasts for one hour and between sessions, patients are expected to practise three times a day and keep a diary of each session. The diary is essential as it provides the trainer with information on the patient's progress, without which training cannot continue.

At the start of the training the patient is shown how to carry out a body check; this simply means making sure they are comfortable, for example, being aware of any tension and trying to let it go and, if sitting in a chair, ensuring that their feet touch the ground. 'Cancelling out' of the exercise is also taught to ensure that the patient can stop whenever he/she wants and is not dependent on the trainer; cancellation is done at the end of each exercise.

The standard exercises are then taught, starting with the heaviness exercise, which is practised by the patient over seven days, before the other exercises are introduced one at a time over the eight weeks. During this time the trainer also adds, where appropriate, intentional exercises; these are cathartic and designed to help the patient deal with emotional problems. In addition, a partial exercise is taught for use outside the standard session whenever the need arises; for example, when experiencing a panic attack.

Two follow-up sessions are held at six weeks and three months after completion of the standard exercises. Patients are advised to contact the trainer during these periods if they have any problems with the method. When first learning the technique a person may experience memories of events long past, such as old injuries. This is normal and occurs only during the exercise; with more experience of the method, it is common to feel heaviness and warmth in the limbs as well as a general feeling of deep relaxation during the exercises.

Stages of technique

Each weekly session consists of the following stages:

- interview/assessment of client
- introduction to autogenic training including body check, cancellation technique and first standard heaviness exercise — dominant arm
- heaviness of arms and legs
- heaviness of neck and shoulders, partial exercise and peace formulae
- warmth of arms and legs plus introduction to intentional exercises
- heart beat
- breathing
- solar plexus
- forehead.

Follow-up sessions are as follows:

- Autogenic training check and introduction to space exercise and personal motivation formulae
- Autogenic training progress check and introduction to organ-specific formulae; advice on the continuation of using the therapy.

Therapeutic potential in nursing

Autogenic training is a unique relaxation technique that can be used in a variety of health care settings both as a preventive and for improving quality of life for those with illness. Its benefits include:

- deep relaxation
- stress reduction
- pain management
- controlling anticipatory nausea/vomiting (in patients undergoing chemotherapy/radiotherapy treatment)
- improving confidence
- controlling/getting rid of panic attacks
- improving sleeping patterns
- integrating awareness of mind and body
- hypertension, etc.

Contraindications for use

Not everyone is suited to autogenic training, in particular:

- children under 5 years
- those with no motivation
- people with a personality disorder
- patients with acute psychoses

In some instances, it is important for the patient to be under medical supervision during the training, notably in cases of:

- unstable epilepsy
- insulin-dependent diabetes
- chronic psychoses.

Those who have used unprescribed drugs (e.g. LSD) may also be unsuitable.

Summary

Autogenic training has great potential for use by nurses, particularly those working in the primary care sector, i.e. Health Visitors/District Nurses/Practice Nurses and nurses involved in caring for patients with chronic/terminal illness. Training to teach the method takes 2 years and applicants must have undertaken autogenic training themselves and become proficient in self-use for at least 3 months after the course (approximately 9 months in total). All applicants must hold a qualification in one of the health care professions, e.g. medicine, nursing. A list of qualified registered therapists is available from The British Association for Autogenic Training and Therapy (BAFATT).

REFERENCES

BAFATT 1993 Autogenic training information leaflet. BAFATT, London
Coleman J 1988 Luthe's cathartic autogenic training: a therapist's handbook. BAFATT, London
Crocker P R, Grozelle C 1991 Journal of Sports Medicine and Physical Fitness 31 (2): 277–282
Freedman R R et al 1991 Psychosomatic medicine. American Psychosomatic Society
Kaufman K L, Olson R, Tarnowski J K 1989 Self-regulation treatment to reduce the aversiveness of cancer chemotherapy. Journal of Adolescent Health Care (USA) 4: 323–327
Luthe W 1963 Journal of the Hillside Hospital, New York 12 (2): 106–121
Luthe W 1970 Autogenic therapy: research and theory. Grune & Stratton, New York, vol 4
Luthe W, Schultz J H 1969 Autogenic therapy. Grune & Stratton, London, vol 1

FURTHER READING — JOURNALS

Crowther D 1991 Complementary therapy in practice. Nursing Standard 5: 25–27
Faulkner A 1990 Autogenics — neighbourhood venture. Nursing Times 86: 50–52
Research in autogenic training is ongoing and has resulted in numerous papers of which abstracts are available in English through the Medline database.

FURTHER READING — BOOKS

Baudouin C 1921 Suggestion and autosuggestion. George Allen & Unwin, London

Kermani K 1990 Autogenic training: the effective holistic way to better health. Souvenir Press, London

Luthe W, Schultz J H 1969 Autogenic therapy. Grune & Stratton, New York, vols 1, 2, 3

Luthe W 1970 Autogenic therapy: dynamics of autogenic neutralisation. Grune & Stratton, New York, vol 5

Luthe W 1973 Autogenic therapy: treatment with autogenic neutralisation. Grune & Stratton, New York, vol 6

Pelletier K P 1982 Mind as healer, mind as slayer: a holistic approach to preventing stress disorders. Allen & Unwin, London, p 227–244

USEFUL ADDRESSES

The registered training body is:

British Association for Autogenic
Training and Therapy (BAFATT)
18 Holtsmere Close
Garston
Watford
Herts WD2 6NG

Centre for Autogenic Training
Wirral Holistic Care Services
St Catherine's Hospital
Church Road
Birkenhead
Wirral L42 OLQ

9 Biofeedback

David Bray

Biofeedback — *a method of training which enables a person, mostly with the help of electronic equipment, to learn to control otherwise involuntary bodily functions* — 'learning to play the internal organs' (Lang 1979).

The word biofeedback has been defined as 'information about the state of biological processes, and is used to describe any technique which increases the ability of a person to voluntarily control physiological activities by being provided with information about those activities' (Olton & Noonberg 1980). Biofeedback mostly uses electronic instruments which, when connected to an individual, can measure, amplify and display involuntary physiological processes on a moment to moment basis (Patel 1988). It works on the basic principle that feedback of information, or knowledge of results, is essential for the efficient learning of any skill. The skill in this instance is the control of a given physiological activity, such as heart rate. The information, or knowledge, is the ongoing level of that activity. By monitoring someone's heart rate, for example, and presenting this information to them in a sensible form, such as a digital display, control of the heart rate can be learned (Hume 1976). If such activity is part of a disorder which is not entirely the result of irreversible organic pathology, the trainee can then learn to change the levels of the activity and restore normal function.

The process of biofeedback can be seen as a feedback loop, as shown in Figure 9.1. The level of activity of a 'target organ' is picked up by an instrument, which produces signals presented to the trainee through the senses (sight, sound or other). These are then interpreted by the trainee at the conscious level (brain). The appropriate state of mind or bodily sensations which either increase or decrease activity levels are then identified and enhanced by the trainee to modify the activity of the target organ. A target organ can be any body part

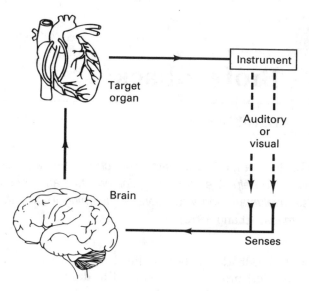

Figure 9.1 *The biofeedback loop.*

from which changing levels of activity can be demonstrated, directly or indirectly, for example skin, muscle, brain, heart, blood vessels, respiratory system. Feedback from a particular target organ is often used to affect other functions; for example in influencing essential hypertension by modifying skin resistance.

HISTORICAL BACKGROUND

For several hundred years, there have been reports from India of yogis who could slow their heart beat, increase their body temperature, survive with little oxygen (reduce their metabolic rate), and influence other bodily functions not normally under voluntary control. However, those capable of this control underwent rigorous and lengthy training, usually in a religious context, and the reports failed to suggest techniques that could be effectively taught to a large percentage of unselected individuals (Barber 1970). More recently, control of involuntary functions has been achieved using hypnosis, autogenic training, and spontaneously in a few rare individuals (Green et al 1970). Using electronic instruments to provide direct readings of levels of involuntary activities has led to a range of effective techniques, representing a synthesis of ancient skills and modern technology.

One of the first recorded successful uses of biofeedback instrumentation was by the Russian psychologist Lisina in 1958, involving taught control of vascular constriction and dilatation (Gatchel & Price 1979). There has been an explosion of research into biofeedback since then, and it is estimated that over 3000 journal articles and 100 books have been published. Many early research findings were disputed due to faulty methodology, but biofeedback is increasingly accepted and Schwartz (1987) suggests it has come of age.

TREATMENT

Biofeedback instruments

These are often called machines but this is not strictly correct, as a machine is something that performs work. However, the instruments used in biofeedback do not *do anything to* people. They are measuring devices, and only provide information about fluctuating activity levels of target organs. In this respect, biofeedback instruments should be seen as teaching aids only, and are no longer needed once the trainee has learned the skill. Instruments are designed according to the target organ activity to be monitored. Any electrical current applied to the skin is not felt by the trainee, and mains-powered equipment has built-in safety features to avoid potentially dangerous direct contact with mains electricity:

- Skin resistance/conductivity monitors (galvanic skin response — GSR; electrodermal response — EDR): register general levels of autonomic arousal; activity increases during 'tension' and reduces during relaxation.

- Skin temperature monitors: register skin temperature changes related to vasodilation/vasoconstriction, which is an indication of the stress response in some people, and is also important in some peripheral vascular disorders. A simplified version is the use of strips or 'dots' of thermoreactive material which adhere to the skin, changing colour with skin temperature changes, e.g. black when tense, blue when relaxed ('Biodots' — see Useful Addresses). Unless the user is properly informed, this material could be very misleading, since some people do not exhibit skin temperature changes when tense, and the environmental temperature must be within a certain constant range when the material is used. Within these limitations, they are useful aids for relaxation training, some peripheral vascular disorders and migraine headaches.

- Myographic (EMG) monitors: provide a direct indication of activity in accessible muscles, and can be used to enhance muscle activity, as in recovery after CVA or to reduce electrical activity in muscles when there is too much activity (muscular tension) in the resting state and bring about effective muscular relaxation
- Electroencephalographic (EEG) monitors: register brain wave activity, enabling trainees to generate wave forms such as alpha waves, associated with a relaxed state. Systems have been designed whereby the desired wave forms enable a model electric train to move round a track.
- Heart/pulse rate or rhythm monitors.

Computer-enhanced biofeedback

Computerized systems are available which enable records to be kept at any stage of the training process, in the form of graphs. These records can be printed out. The computerized system can also make learning more fun. The signal of activity levels is used as a control for computer games. For example, tensing and releasing the frontalis muscle to guide a ship through a channel on the computer screen can help tension headache (Myolink system and Myostart programme, Aleph One Ltd — see Useful Addresses).

The training method

During a biofeedback session, the trainee sits or lies comfortably in relatively quiet surroundings (earphones can be used for auditory feedback, or to reduce distracting background noise). Comfortable electrodes are attached to clean skin. The anatomical location of the electrodes depends on which target organ or type of instrument is used: for general electrodermal response, usually around two fingers; for muscle activity, to the skin near the muscle origin and insertion; for temperature regulation, to the skin of hands or feet; and for EEG activity, to the cranial area. The trainee spends sessions of 15 to 40 minutes practising with the instrument. The total number of sessions needed will vary from person to person, depending upon the nature of the problem, and the degree of compliance (from 4 to 20 sessions). As with training in any kind of skill, there will be individual differences in initial capacities for learning and learning rates. Sessions may take place several times per week and continue from a few weeks to a few months. Once the trainee has been shown what to do, the continued presence of the trainer is not needed, as the trainee continues to learn on their own with the aid of the instrument.

Stages of technique

First contact — explanation. The most important aspect of biofeedback is *learning* on the part of the trainee, who should be well-informed about the concepts, aims and process of training. General considerations are that biofeedback involves the learning of a skill, is not an instant answer, will take time and practice, and that any problems that arise should be recognized and discussed with the trainer. The key factors for success are high motivation and compliance on the part of the trainee.

Initial session/s with the instrument — familiarization. The main aim of the first session is for the trainee to become familiar with the equipment. To most people, biofeedback is a strange and unusual experience and a gradual introduction to the process is sometimes necessary. The trainee finds out how the target organ levels change with alterations in movement, breathing and mental activity. By mutual agreement with the trainer, the trainee is then shown (if necessary) which accessory relaxation techniques, or other methods, to use to enhance the biofeedback process.

Follow-up sessions — practice. Trainees continue to practise on their own. Some briefing or debriefing with the trainer may be needed occasionally.

Completion of training. Training is complete when the trainee is able to self-regulate without the instrumentation.

Therapeutic potential in nursing

Therapeutic benefit depends upon the instruments (and time) available to the nurse, the level of expertise and the environment. The needs of patients in a community clinic differ from those of hospital inpatients. The type of department in a hospital determines which kind of biofeedback is appropriate. For the beginner, a GSR/EDR monitor is perhaps the first step, since it is less expensive, portable, versatile and easily applied. Conscientious reading and study are essential for basic knowledge and further progress. General applications include:

- Demonstrating to patients that tension is related to mental activity, and that they are capable of developing some control of tension levels
- Rapidly and effectively teaching patients to relax/release tension, including enhancing and accelerating the effects of autogenic training, hypnosis, meditation-based relaxation, and progressive

muscular relaxation (biofeedback instruments let trainees know clearly and quickly when they are doing the right thing)

- Pain control

- Observing whether or not an anxious patient (injured, preoperative, prepartum, etc.) is 'calming down'.

Biofeedback can also be used to influence behaviour (see contraindications):

- by reducing anxiety levels in phobic patients

- by assisting in reducing tension as part of weight control and in substance dependency.

It can contribute to the management of specific conditions (but see contraindications) such as:

- asthma

- cardiovascular disorders (arrhythmias, hypertension, recovery from coronary episode)

- headache (migraine and tension)

- insomnia

- neuromuscular problems (rehabilitation, spasticity, paralysis (especially after CVA), muscular tension)

- peripheral vascular disorders.

A prospective biofeedback trainer should (ideally) have the following:

- Some technical ability in order to apply and maintain the instruments

- Good communication, counselling and teaching skills

- Knowledge of a variety of relaxation/stress management techniques which can be used to supplement biofeedback training

- Some ability to understand and control their own stress responses.

Contraindications for use

People who are repelled by instruments/computers (this is also a contraindication for would-be trainers), who see no possibility of having any control over what happens to them, or who have very low self-esteem, are not suitable candidates. The Biofeedback Standards Association's 'Applications, standards and guidelines' (Schwartz & Fehmi 1982) is suggested as essential reading for any prospective trainer and includes the following 'cautions and contraindications':

- A variety of psychiatric disorders, including severe depression

- Impairment of attention/memory, as in dementia or mental handicap

- Anyone experiencing a severe health or emotional crisis
- Low blood pressure
- Seizure disorders
- Extreme scepticism.

Relative contraindications apply when patients are receiving medication for certain conditions such as asthma, glaucoma and diabetes mellitus (Schwartz 1987). The patient's physician should be consulted, and medication doses monitored if biofeedback training is used. Where possible, training should be part of multidisciplinary health care.

Biofeedback training using instrumentation is ideally suited to the busy nurse who may have a reasonable amount of time available to teach self-help techniques to patients. The method enables people to take an active part in their own recovery. It is non-invasive and fosters self-reliance, independence and responsibility for improvement in health.

REFERENCES

Barber T X 1970 In: Stoyva J et al (eds) Biofeedback and self-control. Aldine Atherton, Chicago

Gatchel R J, Price K P (eds) 1979 Clinical applications of biofeedback: appraisal and status. Pergamon, New York

Green E, Green A, Walters M 1970 Voluntary control of internal states: physiological and psychological. In : Stoyva J et al (eds) Biofeedback and self-control. Aldine Atherton, Chicago

Hume W I 1976 Biofeedback. Annual Research Review. Eden Press, Lancaster, vol 2

Lang P J 1979 In: Gatchel R J, Price K P (eds) Clinical applications of biofeedback: appraisal and status. Pergamon, New York

Olton D S, Noonberg A R 1980 Biofeedback — clinical applications in behavioural medicine. Prentice Hall, Englewood Cliffs, New Jersey

Patel C 1988 Biofeedback and self-regulation. In: Rankin-Box D F (ed) Complementary health therapies: a guide for nurses and the caring professions. Croom Helm, Beckenham, Kent

Schwartz M S 1987 Biofeedback — a practitioner's guide. Guilford Press, New York

Schwartz M S, Fehmi L 1982 Applications, standards and guidelines for providers of biofeedback services. Biofeedback Society of America (see AAPB below)

FURTHER READING – JOURNALS

Biofeedback and Self-Regulation — published quarterly by Plenum, New York

Patel C, Marmot M M, Terry D J 1981 Controlled trial of biofeedback-aided behavioural methods in reducing mild hypertension. British Medical Journal 282: 2005–2008

Biofeedback research is published in a wide variety of contexts and lack of space prohibits a detailed list — other journal references can be found in the above references.

FURTHER READING – BOOKS

Basmajian J V 1983 Biofeedback: principles and practice for clinicians. Williams & Wilkins, Baltimore

Brown B 1977 Stress and the art of biofeedback. Harper & Row, New York

Hume W I 1977 Biofeedback. Annual Research Review. Eden Press, Lancaster, vol 2

Stoyva J et al (eds) 1972 on (annuals) Biofeedback and self-control. Aldine Atherton, Chicago

USEFUL ADDRESSES

Because biofeedback instruments do not change patients, but only supply information to encourage people to be self-caring, they are safe and unlikely to cause harm. Currently there is no standardized training in Britain, and no central register. However, the addresses cited here are sources of national information.

Association of Applied
Psychophysiology and Biofeedback
10200 West 44th Ave #304
Wheat Ridge
CO 80033, USA

International Stress Management
Association (UK Branch)
South Bank University
LPSS
103 Borough Rd
London SE1 0AA

British Holistic Medical Association
179 Gloucester Place
London NW1 6DX

Biofeedback instrument suppliers:

Aleph One Ltd
The Old Court House
High Street
Bottisham
Cambridge CB5 9BB
Tel: 01223 811679

(also an excellent source of publications on research and practical applications)

Biodata Ltd
10 Stocks Street
Manchester M8 8QG
Tel: 0161 834 6688

Biodots
Stresswise
Department of Biological Science
Manchester Metropolitan
University
John Dalton Building
Chester Street
Manchester M1 5GD

10 Communication skills and counselling

Elizabeth Evans

Counselling skills — *a repertoire of learnt behaviours, both verbal and non-verbal, which enable a rapport to be established between nurse and client and facilitate communication.*

Communication is an essential component of health care. Nurses communicate with clients, relatives and other health professionals, in a range of settings. Verbal and non-verbal communication is the means to understanding and assessing clients. This is, perhaps, of particular importance in complementary medicine, where the client practitioner relationship is central to the treatment. However, there is much evidence to suggest that nurse/client communication is not always successful (Kagan et al 1986). Research has demonstrated that patients feel dissatisfied with both the quality of communication and the quantity of information received (Ley 1988). What is said to clients is not understood and frequently forgotten (Reading 1981, Taub & Baker 1983).

In an attempt to close this communication gap, skills derived from counselling are increasingly being used in nursing, and should be a part of complementary therapies training. Counselling skills are included in Project 2000 programmes and are a component of many post-registration courses.

One result of the movement away from the medical model of health care, towards a holistic approach, has been an expansion of the nurse's role and subsequent developments in nursing skills. The shift towards complementary therapies emphasizes more direct communication, based on both touch and discussion. Changes within nursing and pressures from present health policies (Health of the Nation 1992), have given greater emphasis to effective communication. Complementary therapies are part of the move towards a lifestyle-approach to health. These, along with individualized patient care, community care, health education and preventive health measures all rely on effective communication by nurses for their success.

There is evidence that counselling skills can enhance the therapeutic relationship enabling growth, change and healing to take place (Truax & Carkhuff 1967). As the effectiveness of interpersonal skills in nursing practice is recognized, training syllabus guidelines are attempting to respond to research findings (Kagan et al 1986).

HISTORICAL BACKGROUND

Historically, counselling draws from a range of theories. These may be broadly divided into:

- Humanistic — Carl Rogers
- Psychoanalytic — Sigmund Freud
- Behavioural — B. F. Skinner.

Although both psychoanalytic and behavioural theories are used in health care, humanistic theory is most appropriate for nursing interventions. Best known of the humanists are Carl Rogers, the founder of client-centred therapy (Rogers 1961) and Eric Berne who developed Transactional Analysis (popularized through books such as *Games People Play* Berne 1964).

Nelson-Jones (1982) suggested the following features common to all approaches:

- An explanation of the theory's underlying assumptions
- An explanation of how individual behaviour was acquired
- An explanation of how the behaviour was perpetuated
- Practical ways in which the behaviour can be changed.

Many theorists have taken an eclectic approach, drawing from the various skills to formulate a model or framework for practice. Such an approach, frequently encountered in health care, is the helping model of Egan (1990). Egan describes the age-old belief that some people are capable of enabling others to cope with the problems of life. Today, this role falls to counsellors, the clergy, psychiatrists and social workers. In addition to these front-line workers, others who come into contact with individuals during times of crisis or transition are expected, complementary to their primary role, to help with personal problems. This last group includes nurses.

As nurses have been increasingly expected to use aspects of counselling in daily practice, it has become important to describe what this entails. There is a difference between professional counselling and the use of the general principles of counselling and much of the nurse/patient relationship falls into the latter category, commonly referred to as 'counselling skills' (Bond 1993). This has been recognized by the British Association of Counselling (BAC 1989) in their code of ethics and practice for counselling skills.

TREATMENT

An awareness of the impact of non-verbal cues is essential in counselling.

Non-verbal communication includes:

- clothing and appearance
- use of paralanguage (meaning conveyed by tone and pitch of voice, such as 'uhhu' or 'hmmm')
- bodily contact and proximity
- respect of personal space
- eye contact
- facial expression.

Generally, counselling skills involve the following:

- accurate listening
- attending
- the use of silence
- appropriate body language
- reflecting, i.e. repeating the client's words to demonstrate listening
- summarizing, i.e. accurately paraphrasing what the client has said
- self-awareness
- use of 'minimal encouragers' or paralanguage.

These skills should be used in a client-centred framework. Rogers (1980) described four core conditions needed to establish a counselling relationship, as follows:

- Empathy
- Genuineness
- Respect
- Unconditional positive regard.

When these core conditions are present, the fundamental counselling relationship exists in which the client may move towards the resolution of problems. In a pure Rogerian framework, the counsellor adopts a non-directive client-centred role. The theory is, that within the therapeutic relationship, clients will be enabled to self-actualize and develop the abilities, latent within themselves, to resolve or accept their situation.

Other models of counselling are problem-centred, rather than client-centred. In these, the skills of problem-solving are used within a framework. For example, Egan (1990) developed a three-stage, helping model that, whilst encompassing Roger's core conditions, is an action model in which the counsellor facilitates the client's progress: at each stage of the model, some form of action is required of the client.

Therapeutic potential in nursing

The interaction between nurse and client is therapeutic (Burnard 1992) and this is particularly pertinent in the practice of complementary therapies. Examples of specific uses of therapeutic communication skills (Burnard 1992) within nursing are as follows:

- Assessment
- Explaining treatments and therapies
- HIV/AIDS counselling
- Genetic counselling; decisions concerning screening
- Grief and bereavement counselling
- To relieve anxiety and stress on admission or discharge
- Selection of a complementary therapy
- Breaking bad news to clients or relatives
- Health education
- Drugs and alcohol counselling
- Mental health care
- Prior to, during and after complementary therapy.

Contraindications for use

Counselling skills should not be used to:

- Relate one's own similar experience
- Moralize
- Psychoanalyse
- Fantasize about what may be the problem

- Persuade or bully
- Satisfy the nurse's curiosity or needs.

Counselling is not an innate skill but requires careful training and the ability to recognize one's own limitations. In the field of complementary therapies the frequently close relationship that may form highlights the need for effective counselling skills. The practitioner should also be aware of the necessity of referring on clients who require specialist help.

Carl Rogers (1980) quotes Lao-tzu:

'If I keep from meddling with people, they take care of themselves,
If I keep from commanding people, they behave themselves,
If I keep from preaching at people, they improve themselves,
If I keep from imposing on people, they become themselves.'

Summary

Whilst not all nurses may see themselves as effective counsellors, effective communication skills are essential in daily nursing practice. The acquisition of skills drawn from counselling broadens the individual nurse's repertoire of skills leading towards improved client care. The therapeutic value of counselling skills is such that they should form an essential part of training.

REFERENCES

Berne E 1964 Games people play. Grove Press, New York

Bond T 1993 Counselling, counselling skills and professional roles. In: Bayne R, Nicolson P (eds) Counselling and psychology for health professionals. Chapman and Hall, London

BAC 1989 Code of ethics and practice for counselling skills. British Association for Counselling (BAC), Rugby

Burnard P 1992 Effective communication skills for health professionals. Chapman and Hall, London

Egan G 1990 The skilled helper: a systematic approach to effective helping, 4th edn. Brooks/Cole, CA, USA

Kagan C, Evans J, Kay B 1986 A manual of interpersonal skills for nurses: an experiential approach. Harper & Row, London

Ley P 1988 Communicating with patients. Chapman and Hall, London

Nelson-Jones R 1982 The theory and practice of counselling psychology. Cassell, London

Orr J 1988 Social skills. In: Rankin-Box D (ed) Complementary health therapies: a guide for nurses and the caring professions. Chapman and Hall, London

Reading A E 1981 Psychological preparations for surgery: patient recall of information. Journal of Psychosomatic Research 25: 57–62

Rogers C R 1961 On becoming a person. Houghton Mifflin, Boston

Rogers C R 1980 A way of being. Houghton Mifflin, Boston

Taub H A, Baker M T 1983 The effect of repeated testing upon comprehension of informed consent materials by elderly volunteers. Experimental Aging Research 9: 135–138

Truax C B, Carkuff R R 1967 Towards effective counselling and psychotherapy. Aldine, Chicago

FURTHER READING – JOURNALS

Bond T 1991 HIV counselling: Report on National Survey and Consultation 1990. BAC/Department of Health, London
A joint study by the Department of Health and the British Association for Counselling. The importance of respect for the client's perspective is emphasized and the potential for role conflict addressed.

Roberts R, Fallowfield L 1990 The goals of cancer counsellors. Journal of the British Association for Counselling 1: 88–91
A study of cancer counsellors found that those holding a qualification in counselling, had a greater commitment to the goal of client self-determination as opposed to organizational or personal goals.

FURTHER READING – BOOKS

Bayne R, Nicolson P (eds) 1993 Counselling and psychology for health professionals. Chapman and Hall, London
A collection of topics related to counselling by experts in the field. Of particular interest to nurses are chapters on AIDS counselling, the needs of sexually abused children and gender issues in ageing. The chapter by Bond clearly explains the role of counselling skills within health care. There is a useful section on research and evaluation.

Burnard P 1992 Effective communication skills for health professionals. Chapman and Hall, London
Wide-ranging suggestions for ways to improve communication. Includes teaching, computing and presentation skills, in addition to counselling. The second section looks particularly at the therapeutic skills of listening and counselling.

Nelson-Jones R 1982 The theory and practice of counselling psychology. Cassell, London
A detailed description of the major theories underlying counselling. Relates theory to counselling practice and includes exercises for students.

Stewart W 1992 An A–Z of counselling theory and practice. Chapman and Hall, London

An alphabetical coverage of terms and concepts related to counselling.
Concise, yet in enough depth to aid understanding. As the author says
'a handy reference book'.

USEFUL ADDRESSES

Listed below are organizations which either offer counselling training or are
useful reference points for particular client groups. Some, such as Relate,
cover both areas.

Alcoholics Anonymous
PO Box 1
Stonebow House
Stonebow
York
YO1 2NJ

BACUP (British Association of
Cancer United Patients)
3 Bath Place
Rivington Street
London
EC2A 3JR

British Association for Counselling
37a Sheep Street
Rugby
Warwickshire
CV21 3BX

Centre for Counselling and
Psychotherapy Education
21 Lancaster Rd
London
W11 1QL

Childline
Freepost 1111
London
W1H 0BR

CRUSE
126 Sheen Rd
Richmond
TW9 1UR

MIND
The White Building
Fitzalan Square
Sheffield
S1 2AY

Relate
Herbert Gray College
Little Church Street
Rugby
Warwickshire
CV21 3AP

11 Healing

Denise Rankin-Box

Healing — *the practice of a conscious intentionality to improve health and well-being.*

Healing may take many forms, such as faith healing, the 'laying on of hands' or ritual Shamanism, and is one of the oldest and most widespread forms of health care. Even today it is highly sought after, as reflected by the estimated number (over 20 000) of healers practising in the UK (Fulder & Monroe 1981, Turton 1988). Benor (1991) reported 8000 healers were registered in 16 different organizations in the UK and working under a unified code of conduct; these organizations also provide formal instruction in healing.

Alongside the reductionist approach of conventional medicine health care, religious or spiritual healing beliefs and practices seem to be flourishing (Glik 1990). There is also a growing body of literature on the origins of healing and healing belief systems (Easthope 1985, Benor 1990, Glik 1990, Graham 1991). Amongst the many terms used to refer to healing are 'faith', 'spiritual', 'psychic', 'paranormal' and 'shamanistic' (Benor 1990). The 'shaman – scientist' (Achterberg 1985) is attempting to link ancient intuitive practices and modern medicine. Perhaps new health care models will look to the original Hippocratic model of 2000 years ago which held that — 'there is one flow; one common breathing; all things are in sympathy' (Graham 1991).

There are many forms of healing and only those most commonly encountered can be described here. Two features that these different practices have in common are:

- close links with a belief system which may be religious, spiritual, social or cultural
- the belief that healers channel healing 'energy' to the client.

A healing session usually involves assessment of the client's energy field and the passage of energy to them through the healer by gentle touch or a light sweeping of the healer's hands near the client's body. In addition, more complex rituals may be used. Healers may also treat by distant healing, using thought, intent, meditation or prayer to project healing to a client who may be some distance away (Benor 1991).

Healing has been performed safely in the clinical setting and particular forms seem to be effective for pain relief, relaxation and in promoting wound healing and reducing post-operative pain (Beutler et al 1988, Wirth et al 1993a, b). Clearly, healing should not be performed without the client's consent and ideally the form used should be in accordance with their own beliefs.

HISTORICAL BACKGROUND

The sheer diversity of healing practices and the belief systems from which they arise makes it difficult to provide a general history. Archaeological and anthropological evidence suggests that healing is rooted in ancient shamanistic practices, linked to magic and mystery (Achterberg 1985, Graham 1986, 1991). Mystic tradition views the universe or cosmos as 'one'; everything is interrelated (including people). A mystic/healer may have an enhanced perception of this universe and, along with heightened sensitivity and awareness, uses certain rituals to interpret and work with the universal forces.

Shamanism is commonly attributed to the Tungus, Siberian tribes, but shamanistic methods seem to have been in use as far back as 20 000 years. Shaman healers were engaged in maintaining the harmony both of individuals and of the tribe. They were considered to have certain powers aligned with the natural forces of the environment; they had a knowledge of plants and herbs, were skilled in healing rituals and were able to communicate with the spirits. The shaman was an holistic practitioner, attempting to harmonize individual and environment.

In ancient Greece, the life-force was perceived as being in a state of dynamic harmony (Graham 1991). Any problems, such as illness, were due to disharmony affecting the life-force. Similarly, Egyptian medicine considered the condition of the whole person, although there were different healers for different problems. Hippocrates' approach to health care also focused on harmony. He emphasized nature's healing power — the vix medicatrix (Graham 1991) — and his students studied the effects of the seasons and the elements on health in a model not dissimilar to that of traditional Chinese medicine.

In the early fourteenth century, climatic changes resulted in crop failures and starvation across Europe. Together with unhygienic living conditions, this led to the spread of the disease Black Death which wiped out up to one half of Europe's population. The survival rate of women was seven times that of men and many believed that women were using some form of magic not only to survive but also to kill men (Achterberg 1990). The rise of Christianity in Europe directly influenced the practice of healing which was claimed as the exclusive domain of the church (Turton 1988). Women healers continued to function under the close eye of the church but, by the late 1300s, women were banned from officially training in medicine and it was then claimed that they must have acquired their knowledge from the devil. The churches' position was 'that if a woman dare to cure without having studied, she is a witch and must die' (Michelet 1939). Any woman practising healing outside the auspices of the church was subject to extreme persecution and many were labelled witches and burnt at the stake (Turton 1988). As a result, any knowledge of healing practices of the time can only be deduced from records of witchcraft trials (Graham 1991).

Despite these controls, the practice of healing continued. One notable healer was Valentine Greatrakes whose healing powers were in considerable demand in the 1700s (Harvey 1983, Turton 1988). Greatrakes was one of the first healers to invite scientific scrutiny of his work (Turton 1988). At this time, women were still being burnt at the stake for similar healing practices. The antagonism between church and lay healers continued and as recently as 1951 it was still theoretically possible to be arrested under the Witchcraft Act which held the death penalty (MacManaway & Turcan 1983).

TREATMENT

There are an increasing number of studies that demonstrate the positive effects of particular forms of healing, and indeed Benor (1990), when reviewing research on spiritual healing, commented that if healing were a drug it would be accepted as effective on the basis of current research results. Healing can be of benefit in a number of clinical settings. Benor (1990) reviewed 131 controlled trials of healing and concluded that 56 of these demonstrated a positive effect. A few of the many forms of healing are described next.

Lay healing — many healers claim to have no specific religious faith or beliefs influencing the healing process. There is usually some concept of rebalancing the client's energy or of the flow of energy between practitioner and client. A range of gentle techniques may be used during the healing experience and healing may also be conducted at a distance.

Spiritual healing — the laying on of hands or healing by prayer/meditation in which a special state of mind is required for healing to occur (Benor 1990). Spiritual healing is closely linked to a belief or faith system. The healer seeks to act as a channel for spiritual energy to flow through to the client. This may occur directly or from a distance.

Reiki — an interactive approach where healing energy is transferred from healer to client. The aim is to restore balance in the client's energy field (Wirth et al 1993a). A range of techniques may be used during healing, such as visualization and the laying on of hands.

LeShan — this technique is not based on an energy theory but advocates that the healer attains an enhanced state of consciousness in order for a 'flow process reality' to occur (Wirth et al 1993). LeShan believed that everyone has a natural ability for healing which can be accessed using the appropriate technique (LeShan 1974, Wirth et al 1993).

Shamanism — this generally refers to specific tribes engaged in maintaining the psychic and ecological equilibrium of their existence (Graham 1991). The shaman's healing powers rely on intuition and interpretation of images. They involve an enhanced state of consciousness induced by using stimulants, rhythmic swaying or other movement, meditation or chanting. Various forms have been described in Polynesia, China, Africa, South Pacific and the Americas (Graham 1991).

Stages of technique

Healing can occur in a special centre, at home or at a distance. A session may last from a few minutes to an hour and several sessions may be needed over a period of time. The client might be treated sitting or lying down. The stages of treatment are usually as follows:

Centring — initial preparation in which the healer becomes relaxed, calm and focused on the care about to be given.

Assessment — the healer may pass his/her hands quickly over the body or head, not usually touching the skin. Temperature changes may be identified by the healer, indicating imbalances of energy.

Healing — stroking or sweeping gestures may be used to balance the client's energy field. Conversely a holding technique may be used on or around the client's body in an attempt to direct energy. Prayers or words may be spoken.

Healing is generally a soothing, gentle experience and clients may experience tingling sensations or temperature changes.

Therapeutic potential in nursing

The possible applications of healing in nursing practice include:

- post-operative pain (dental) (Wirth et al 1993a)
- wound healing (Wirth et al 1990b)
- relaxation
- tension headaches
- anxiety
- hypertension.

Healing does not generally cure but it may initiate a positive process of change.

Contraindications for use

- There appear to be minimal side-effects; occasionally a sensation of light-headedness or faintness may occur.
- It is most important that the client is a willing participant, particularly for methods based on cultural and spiritual belief systems.

Summary

Healing is a gentle, non-invasive form of care that commonly instils feelings of relaxation and calmness (Vickers 1993). It does not require any equipment apart from the healer's hands, one of the key forms of communication at a nurse's disposal (Turton 1988). Healing offers a means of caring for clients in a personal way and may be particularly suited to nursing practice.

REFERENCES

Achterberg J 1985 Imagery in healing. Shamanism and modern medicine. New Science Library, Boston

Achterberg J 1990 Woman as healer. Rider Random Century, London

Benor D J 1990 Survey of spiritual healing research. Complementary Medical Research 4: 9–33

Benor D J 1991 Spiritual healing in clinical practice. Nursing Times 87: 35–37

Beutler J, Attevelt J, Schouten S, Faber J, Mees E, Geuskes G 1988 Paranormal healing and hypertension. British Medical Journal 230: 1491–1494

Easthope G 1985 Three marginal healers. In: Jones K (ed) Sickness and sectarianism. Gower, London

Fulder S J, Monroe R 1981 The status of complementary medicine in the UK. Threshold Foundation

Glik D C 1990 The redefinition of the situation in the social construction of spiritual healing experiences. Sociology of Health and Illness 12: 151–168

Graham H 1986 The human face of psychology. Humanistic psychology in its historical, social and cultural context. Open University Press, Milton Keynes

Graham H 1991 The return of the Shaman: the emergence of a biophysical approach to health and healing. Complementary Medical Research 5 (3): 165–171

Harvey D 1983 The power to heal. An investigation of healing and the healing experience. Aquarian Press, London

LeShan L 1974 The medium, the mystic and the physicist: towards a general theory of the paranormal. Viking Press, New York

MacManaway B, Turcan J 1983 Healing. Thorsons, Wellingborough

Michelet J 1939 Satanism and witchcraft. Translated by Allinson W R 1860 (Secaucas N J: Citadel 1939). Cited in Achterberg J 1990 Woman as healer. Rider Random Century, London

Turton P 1988 Healing: Therapeutic Touch. In: Rankin-Box D F (ed) Complementary health therapies: a guide for nurses and the caring professions. Croom Helm, Beckenham

Vickers A 1993 Complementary medicine and disability: alternatives for people with disabling conditions. Chapman and Hall, London

Wirth D P, Brenlan D R, Levine R J, Rodriguez C M 1993a The effect of complementary healing therapy on postoperative pain after surgical removal of impacted third molar teeth. Complementary Therapies in Medicine 1: 133–138

Wirth D P, Richardson J T, Eidelman W C, O'Malley A C 1993b Full thickness dermal wounds treated with non-contact Therapeutic Touch: a replication and extension. Complementary Therapies in Medicine 1: 127–132

USEFUL ADDRESSES

British Alliance of Healing
Associations
26 Highfield Avenue
Herne Bay
Kent CT6 6LM
Tel: 01227 3738 04

Confederation of Healing
Organisations
25 Ducane Court
London SW17 7JQ

Greater World Christian Spiritual
Association
3 Conway Street
Fitzrovia
London W1P 5HA
Tel: 0171 436 7555

National Federation of Spiritual
Healers
Old Manor Farm Studio
Sunbury-on-Thames
Middlesex TW16 6RG
Tel: 01932 783164

Westbank Healing and Teaching Centre
Strathmiglo
Fife
Scotland KY14 7QP

World Federation of Healing
6 Whitworth House
Buckhurst House
Bexhill-on-Sea
East Sussex TN40 1UA
Tel: 01424 214457

12 Herbal medicine

Helen Busby

Herbal medicine — *the use of whole plant material by trained practitioners to promote recovery from disease and to enable healing to take place.*

Herbalists treat a wide range of conditions, similar to those with which people present to their General Practitioners. Patients of all ages, including infants and pregnant women, can be safely treated with herbs by a qualified experienced practitioner.

Many people use herbal medicine as a treatment of choice (Sharma 1992). Older people, in particular, may continue a long-held allegiance to herbal remedies, and an increasing number of parents see herbal medicine as a gentle first recourse for their children. However, many people turn to a herbalist only after conventional approaches have proved less than satisfactory for their particular condition. This may still be beneficial since herbal treatment is particularly valuable in promoting recovery from various complex conditions.

In an international context, the World Health Organization has recognized the considerable importance of herbal medicine to meeting health needs (WHO 1978). In the UK, the role of the professional herbalist was recognized in the 1968 Medicines Act, which makes provision for particularly potent herbal medicines that are not permitted for over-the-counter sale to be prescribed by a professional herbalist. The National Institute of Medical Herbalists (NIMH), founded in 1864, now oversees standards of practice and ensures high standards of training.

Herbal medicine is at present little used within nursing in the UK, with the exception of the external use of essential oils from herbs for massage (aromatherapy). In European countries such as France and Germany, where herbal medicine is more integrated into the health care system, it is usually the physician who has the responsibility for prescribing the herbs. It is suggested then, that it is the traditional divisions of labour and roles between nurses and physicians, rather than any lack of therapeutic potential, which are primarily responsible for the limited use of herbal medicine within nursing. This challenge to conventional roles will need to be addressed before the therapeutic potential of herbal medicine is likely to be fulfilled. There are a number of small projects, particularly in the area of drug and alcohol dependence, where nurses with additional specialized training in herbal medicine are able to use these skills with their patients.

The practice of herbal medicine requires substantial training (currently 4 years full-time or equivalent part-time) and the therapy is, in the British Medical Association's words, a 'discrete clinical entity' (BMA 1993) rather than a set of techniques.

HISTORICAL BACKGROUND

Herbal medicine has been at the core of most systems of medicine throughout history. Historical sources, including herbals, provide us with information about traditions and systems of herbal medicines from at least the first century BC in ancient Greek, Egyptian and Chinese cultures. However, mythologies suggest, and archaeological findings confirm, that use of herbal medicine began many thousands of years earlier (Griggs 1981). An account by Theophrastus of the medicinal uses of 455 plants, written in the third century BC, was probably the earliest Western herbal. The advent of printing in the sixteenth and seventeenth centuries made it possible for herbals like Culpeper's, published in 1652, to have a wide circulation.

Today, about a quarter of pharmaceutical preparations contain at least one active constituent extracted from plant sources (Farnsworth 1981). Well-known examples among the thousands of drugs originally discovered from plants include digitalis (from Foxglove), aspirin (from Willow and Meadowsweet) and ephedrine (from the Chinese Ephedra).

TREATMENT

A key to herbal treatment is the emphasis on the 'vital force' or life energy of the patient, and mobilizing the self-healing or homoeostatic powers of the body. One implication of this is that the patient's subjective experience of their symptoms is central to the diagnostic process. A detailed case history will be taken as part of the initial consultation, including information that will help the herbalist to assess the personal and social context of an individual's illness or disease. A Western herbalist will use a similar system of diagnosis to current orthodox medicine, with particular emphasis on aetiology.

A herbalist will choose from plants which have general actions, including relaxant, tonic, enhancement of immune resistance, or more specific actions, such as vasodilatory, hypotensive, anti-inflammatory, expectorant and diuretic (Weiss 1988). Different constituents of a prescription or within a single plant combine to form a total effect which is 'more than the sum of the parts', known as synergy. For example, the anti-inflammatory action of the aspirin-like salicylates in Meadowsweet is buffered by a range of other constituents which soothe and protect the mucosa of the digestive tract, making use of the total plant material safer than its chemical counterpart.

Herbs are precribed in a number of forms:

- infusions (herb teas)
- decoctions (roots or barks simmered in water)
- tinctures (concentrated extracts of a herb in a solution of water and alcohol)
- juices
- capsules
- external applications, such as creams, lotions or poultices.

The length of treatment varies according to individual need, but as with many therapies, chronic problems generally take several months, whilst acute problems, even if more severe, are likely to respond in a matter of days or weeks.

Therapeutic potential

Herbal medicine can be effective for a wide range of health problems. Some examples are:

- Vasodilatory (Weiss 1988)
- Cardiovascular system (Ernest 1987)
- Migraines (Murphy et al)
- Anti-inflammatory (Weiss 1988)
- Skin conditions (Sheehan et al 1992)

Contraindications for use

There are few absolute contraindications for the use of herbal medicine by trained practitioners. Contrary to popular belief, not all herbs are safe in all situations. For example:

- Liquorice is not recommended for long-term use by people with hypertension
- Ginseng should not be taken by a person with significant levels of anxiety, tension or restlessness or when there is acute inflammation.

Some conditions associated with organic damage are unlikely to respond to treatment with herbal medicine:

- Certain specific conditions, for example epilepsy, cannot be effectively treated with herbs
- In some cases, such as severe mental illness or distress, herbal treatment could be supportive only in conjunction with appropriate support from a mental health team.

In some conditions, another therapy will be the treatment of choice. For example, insulin-dependent diabetes is best managed by an orthodox physician and some musculoskeletal conditions should be referred for treatment by an osteopath.

Interactions between herbal medicines and other prescribed medicines are possible, for example:

- The trained herbalist would avoid the use of Ephedra with monoamine oxidase inhibitors (MAOIs)
- Some herbs containing cardioactive glycosides, such as Lily of the Valley, would not be prescribed in conjunction with digitalis as they could potentiate each other.

Appropriate use and dosage of herbs, prescribed by trained herbalists, is the key to safety.

Summary

Herbal medicine has a wide range of applications within health care and has a well established historic ancestry. It can be a gentle and highly effective system of health care. Although herbal medicine is currently little used in nursing practice, nurses should be familiar with its use and if giving advice to patients, should ensure they are competent to do so. Herbal medicine should only be prescribed by trained herbalists.

REFERENCES

BMA 1993 Complementary medicines: new approaches to good practice. British Medical Association/Oxford University Press, Oxford

Ernest E 1987 Cardiovascular effects of garlic: a review. Pharmathopeutica 5: 83–89

Farnsworth N 1981 Foreword to Griggs B Green pharmacy: a history of herbal medicine. Jill Norman and Hobhouse, London

Griggs B 1981 Green pharmacy: a history of herbal medicine. Jill Norman and Hobhouse, London

Murphy J J et al 1988 Randomised double-blind placebo-controlled trial of Feverfew in migraine prevention. Lancet ii: 189–192

Sharma U 1992 Complementary medicine today: practitioners and patients. Tavistock/Routledge, London (Chapter 1 contains an overview of some recent surveys of the extent of use of specified complementary medicines)

Sheehan M P et al 1992 Efficacy of traditional Chinese herbal therapy in adult atopic dermatitis. Lancet 340: 13–17

Weiss R F (trans. by Meuss A R) 1988 Herbal medicine. Beaconsfield, Beaconsfield

WHO 1978 The promotion and development of traditional medicine. World Health Organization (WHO) technical report series No. 662. WHO, Geneva

FURTHER READING – RESEARCH

Pharmacologically orientated research is the most extensively published; examples include:

Bradley P (ed) 1992 British herbal compendium, vol 1. A handbook of scientific information on widely used plant drugs. BHMA, Bournemouth

Bradley provides an up-to-date summary of the scientific information available on the chemical constituents of each herb. There is also some information on therapeutic indications, but only in so far as they can be scientifically validated. This points to the research now needed to support and clarify the empirical knowledge that herbalists have.

Farnsworth N R, Kaas C J 1981 An approach utilising information from traditional medicine to identify tumour inhibiting plants. Journal of Ethnopharmacology 3: 85–99

An example of the work being done by ethnobotanists to preserve some of the heritage of empirical knowledge of healing with plants.

Mills S 1991 Herbal medicines: research strategies. Complementary Medical Research 5: 29–35

In this concise review of particular criteria for research into the efficacy of herbal medicines which is relevant and valid, a range of methodologies are considered.

Weiss R F 1988 (trans. by Meuss A R) Herbal medicine. Beaconsfield, Beaconsfield
A careful balance of the old and the new and a review of much pertinent research on traditional uses of herbal medicines by a German physician.

Some examples of clinical research are as follows:

European Journal of Herbal Medicine
This journal has a commitment to publishing a range of research, including clinical. It is affiliated to the National Institute of Medical Herbalists.

The use of uniform formulae instead of individualized treatment in trials of the kind described by Murphy et al and Sheehan et al (above) is, however, likely to lead to less effective treatment.

FURTHER READING – BOOKS

Fulder S 1990 The Tao of medicine: ginseng and other Chinese herbs for inner equilibrium and immune power. Healing Arts Press, Vermont
Hoffmann D 1990 The new holistic herbal. Element Books, Dorset
Weiss R F 1988 (trans. by Meuss A R) Herbal medicine. Beaconsfield, Beaconsfield

USEFUL ADDRESSES

National Institute of Medical Herbalists
9 Palace Gate
Exeter
Devon
Tel: 01392 426022

The main body concerned with representing professional herbal practitioners in the UK and Europe. NIMH will provide lists of qualified practitioners of Western herbal medicine on request or other further information; also subscriptions for the affiliated European Journal of Herbal Medicine.

Register of Chinese Herbal Medicine
PO Box 400
Wembley
Middlesex HA9 9NZ
Tel: 0181 904 1357

Centre of Complementary Health Studies
The University of Exeter
Streatham Court
Rennes Drive
Exeter EX4 4PU

Provides the facility, EXTRACT — database and searches about herbal medicines.

Greenfiles
138 Oak Tree Lane
Mansfield
Nottinghamshire N18 3HR

Produces a quarterly newsletter of research abstracts primarily for holistic herbal practitioners to keep up to date with new developments.

School of Herbal Medicine (Phytotherapy)
Bucksteep Manor
Bodle Street Green
Near Hailsham
East Sussex

The first degree course in herbal medicine at a UK university is planned to be offered from October 1994. Contact National Institute of Medical Herbalists (NIMH) for information.

13 Homoeopathy

Kenneth Atherton

Homoeopathy — *a 200-year-old system of medicine (Haehl 1985) based on the Law of Similars (let like be cured by like). The principle of homoeopathy can be illustrated as follows: within seconds of being stung by the common garden nettle, a red, blotchy and often itchy rash appears. Yet the same nettle can be used to produce a homoeopathic remedy which may stimulate the body's own capacity to heal itself by producing an opposite curative effect. Also, shell fish allergies or generalized urticaria may well respond to a homoeopathic medicine made from the nettle, because although the causes differ the characteristics of the complaint are 'similar'.*

Homoeopathic medicines or remedies are produced from various natural sources — plants, metals, minerals, venoms and stings, and also bacteria or human tissue; for example, extracts of the plant Belladonna (Deadly Nightshade), calcium carbonate (a layer of the oyster shell), lachesis (the venom of the deadly Bushmaster Snake) and bacteria such as *Pneumococcus* (Boericke 1987).

Effectivity results from the process by which remedies are made. The original substances are normally diluted many times in a water and alcohol base. At each dilution, the mixture is shaken vigorously, a process known as 'succussion', which homoeopaths believe gives the final product its power to heal (Livingston 1991). Recent research by the French scientist Jacques Benveniste of the South Paris University suggests that the water/alcohol solution retains the memory of its original substance. Benveniste (1988) reported degranulation of basophils and histamine release when exposed to anti-IgE antibodies at dilutions that were so great that not one single molecule of anti-IgE was present (Benveniste 1988). Dr David Taylor-Reilly of the Glasgow Homoeopathic Hospital compares this phenomenon to the ability of water to form many thousands of variations of snowflake shape. It is suggested that this 'memory' could be the underlying mechanism of homoeopathy (Benveniste 1988).

Potencies are obtained according to accepted pharmaceutical principles. There are two forms of dilution, decimal and centesimal, successive methods of reduction being in steps of 1/10 and 1/100 respectively. The number of stages determines the potency of the dilution or trituration obtained as shown in the table:

Dilution	Concentration		Decimal scale	Centesimal scale
1/10	10%	10^{-1}	D1 or 1×	
1/100	1%	10^{-2}	D2 or 2×	1c or 1cH 1/100
1/1000	0.1%	10^{-3}	D3 or 3×	
1/10000	0.01%	10^{-4}	D4 or 4×	2c or 2cH 1/10000
1/100000	0.001%	10^{-5}	D5 or 5×	
1/1000000	0.0001%	10^{-6}	D6 or 6×	3c or 3cH 1/1000000
1/10		10^{-12}	D12 or 12×	6c or 6cH 1/10
		10^{-18}		9c 1/10
		10^{-24}		12c 1/10
		10^{-60}		30c 1/10
				200c
				1000c or 1M

Homoeopathic medicines are dispensed in four forms depending on the type of prescription:

- powders
- granules
- tablets
- liquids.

The following two examples illustrate prescribing techniques. In the case of powders, it is usual only to medicate the first two or three and follow with a series of unmedicated ones. The reason for this is to allow the medicated part of the prescription time to act. The therapeutic response varies in patients and may take several days to several weeks. Generally this type of prescription is written as follows:

Arsen Alb 1M 1–3   Arsen alb 30 in powders 1 to 3
S.L.12 t.d.s., p.c.   Lactose powders 4 to 12
                                   One powder to be taken dry on the tongue
                                   three times a day after meals in the order
                                   numbered; 4 days' supply

Prescribing habits differ and sometimes a low potency may be given over a course of weeks or months. In these cases, tablets are often used. The tablets are composed of lactose with an added amount of pure sugar. The desired potency of the homoeopathic medicine is absorbed into each tablet. An example of a prescription for tablets is as follows:

Gelsemium 6c 7 g (50 tablets)
1 t.d.s.

Most pharmacies instruct patients undertaking homoeopathic treatment to avoid coffee, peppermint or menthol, as these substances are considered to counteract the effect of the remedies. Homoeopathic medicines in low potencies are readily available over the counter and it is commonplace now to see such preparations in pharmacies and health food shops. These medicines are generally available to the public for self-treatment; for example, Rhus Tox 6c for rheumatism or Chammomilla 6c for teething problems. However, for complex or chronic conditions, a skilled assessment and prescription is often necessary for which a qualified practitioner should be consulted.

Critics have for many years attributed successful homoeopathic treatment to the 'placebo' effect. However, the growing amount of animal research would suggest otherwise. Veterinary surgeon, Christopher Day, carried out a double-blind trial in 1988 on mastitis in cows. The cows were split into two groups and treated over a 12-month period. Group A received a placebo in the form of untreated liquid drops added to the drinking water while for Group B liquid drops containing a homoeopathic medicine were used. The results showed that the cows treated by homoeopathy substantially improved and had fewer relapses than those given the placebo (Day 1988).

Homoeopathy is complementary to conventional medicine, and may be particularly helpful in the alleviation of chronic ailments without the risk of side effects (Koehler 1986).

Training

Presently, under Common Law, non-medically qualified people can set themselves up as homoeopaths and many people without a medical or nursing background have taken courses. These courses often extend over 5 years on a part-time basis and award a qualification which as yet has no statutory recognition. Many lay colleges are striving to achieve good training standards and some turn out excellent homoeopaths. However, it has been suggested that the lack of a medical background and practical hospital experience may be disadvantageous for lay practitioners. Also, a non-medically qualified homoeopath might be less likely to know when to refer a patient for conventional medical opinion (Faculty of Homoeopathy 1993).

The Faculty of Homoeopathy at the Royal London Homoeopathic Hospital, Great Ormond Street, London, is the only statutory recognized training body (Act of Parliament 1950) and in 1993 made educational history by being the first professional training organization to have an MSc degree in Homoeopathic Medicine accredited at a British university. The degree course which started autumn 1994 is at present only open to medical doctors but trained nurses, midwives and pharmacists may complete the first module and be awarded a Certificate in Homoeopathic Medicine.

HISTORICAL BACKGROUND

The dominant name in the history of homoeopathy is that of Hahnemann. The son of a porcelain painter of the Meissen factory in Saxony, Samuel Hahnemann (1755–1843) was a skilled linguist and translator before becoming a chemist and later a physician at the age of 24. It was while translating the Materia Medica of Professor Cullen of Edinburgh that Hahnemann realized the significance of homoeopathic principles.

Hahnemann's first experiments involved the effects of quinine (Chinchona bark), reputed to cure malaria. The resemblance between the effects of quinine and the effects of malaria itself seemed to him more than coincidence (Livingston 1991). Hahnemann self-prescribed repeated doses of pure quinine and developed symptoms similar to those of malaria. He found that dilutions of the drug prepared in a homoeopathic way were effective in curing malaria. Subsequently, many substances were tested on healthy volunteers to determine the symptoms they could produce and so cure. This form of experimentation is known as 'proving'. Hahnemann's methods and teachings were not without their critics but his reputation spread widely. When towards the end of his life he moved to Paris, people waited in their carriages for days in order to consult him.

A post-graduate school of homoeopathy was established late in the nineteenth century in Philadelphia, USA (Tyler-Kent 1979). Homoeopathic hospitals developed in various major cities throughout the UK, including London, Liverpool, Glasgow, Bristol and Tunbridge Wells. Many of these hospitals still exist and are fully recognized under the NHS, patients being referred in the usual way through their GP. All these hospitals are staffed by qualified medical doctors who have undertaken further post-graduate training in homoeopathic medicine.

TREATMENT

No condition, no matter how serious or trivial, is beyond homoeopathic consideration. In advanced stages of terminal illness, substantial pain relief and comfort may be attained. The homoeopathic approach to treatment differs from the conventional. Hahnemann was explicit about how a case history should be recorded and warned against the practitioner being biased or not allowing patients time to describe their symptoms (Koehler 1986). Every symptom is noted as described by the patient, accompanied by the practitioner's observations. Factors possibly considered of little importance conventionally can in homoeopathy be crucial in the choice of a remedy. For example, although two people may present with a similar painful joint, one may report it worse during mobility and the other worse for rest; each would receive a completely different remedy. The choice of any remedy is always based on the totality of the symptoms (Livingston 1991).

A homoeopath will often enquire about the patient's preferences, such as whether they feel more comfortable in a hot or cold environment, whether they have a desire or aversion for sweet foods, salt, condiments, fruit, eggs, fat, cheese or meat. All this information influences the choice of the correct remedy (Agrawal 1980). Questions about general health, sleep, bowel habits, childhood illnesses, alcohol and tobacco intake, family history and, most importantly, the patient's psychological condition will all contribute to the final decision regarding treatment (Boyd 1981). Routine investigations such as temperature, pulse, respiration, blood pressure, weight and laboratory tests are performed as necessary.

Therapeutic potential in nursing

Nurses trained in homoeopathy as a first aid could contribute a great deal to nursing practice. Homoeopathy has much to offer in community care, day nursing, industry, midwifery and nursing homes. It would also be useful in Accident and Emergency Departments, intensive care and medical and surgical units, provided the appropriate authorization is obtained.

Some acute complaints that can be treated are as follows:

- Accident and emergency
  sudden collapse — Carbo Veg
  acute injuries — Arnica
  Injured nerves — Hypericum

- Bites and stings
  wasps or bees — Apis Mel, Urtica Urens, Ledum

- Burns and scalds
  severe blistering — Cantharis
  sunburn — Belladonna
  local application — Calendula

- Care of the chronically and terminally ill, including pain management
  and emotional distress
  terminal illness with restlessness — Arsen Alb
  pains associated with tumours — Euphorbium
  distressed relatives — Gelsemium, Ignatia

- Chemotherapy and radiotherapy — to assist with nausea and
  general health
  skin tenderness after radiotherapy — Cantharis

- Community care — with a wide application for district nursing in the
  treatment of wounds and leg ulcers and care of the elderly
  post-operative wounds — Arnica, Staphysagria
  leg ulcers — Calendula, Flouric Acid

- Coughs, colds, sore throats and influenza
  influenza — Gelsemium, Aconite
  fever — Belladonna
  coughs — Bryonia

- Distressed relatives, e.g. shock and grief reactions
  shock — Gelsemium, Aconite
  grief — Ignatia

- Endoscopic procedures
  pre-general anaesthetic — Phosphorus
  apprehensive patients — Gelsemium, Argentum Nitrate

- First aid — road traffic accidents, including air, sea and mountain
  rescue (as for accident and emergency)

- Hayfever and simple allergies — Homoeopathic Grass Pollen,
  Allium Cepa

- Hyperactive children — Belladonna, Agaricus

- Insomnia — Coffea

- Midwifery (pre- and post-natal care)
  miscarriage prevention — Caulophyllum
  injuries associated with childbirth — Arnica, Staphysagria

- Pre- and post-surgical management including dental surgery
  before any surgical procedure — Arnica

- Stress and phobias — including anticipation and fear of unpleasant investigations and surgical procedures
  phobic states — Phosphorus, Argentum Nitrate
  anticipatory fear — Gelsemium.

Contraindications for use

On the whole, homoeopathic treatment is safe and will not interfere with conventional medicines prescribed by the patient's GP. However, some homoeopaths feel that treatment may be less effective if combined with drugs, particularly steroid preparations.

Contraindications are few but the following categories are important:

- Patients known to have sensitivity to milk products should inform their homoeopath as lactose is often used as a tablet base for the homoeopathic remedy. Remedies can then be supplied in a water and alcohol base in the form of drops.

- Diabetic patients should inform the homoeopath of their condition because of the lactose based medication. An alternative non-sugar based medication can be used.

- Young babies may not be able to metabolize alcohol, so remedies should be alcohol free. Alcohol-free medicine may be dissolved in a little water and administered via the feeding bottle.

- Where possible homoeopaths should collaborate with medical colleagues and never attempt to treat a patient with a serious illness whose diagnosis is uncertain without prior consultation with the patient's GP.

Summary

Homoeopathy can be surprisingly effective but patients must be prepared to give the treatment time to achieve a therapeutic response. This sometimes means a change in lifestyle, which could include an alteration in diet, more relaxation and exercise to complement the treatment.

REFERENCES

Agrawal V R 1980 A repertory of desires and aversions. Vijay, Delhi
Benveniste J 1988 Human basophil degranulation triggered by very dilute anti serum against IgE. Nature 333: 816–818

Boericke W 1987 Homoeopathic materia medica with repertory. Homoeopathic Book Service, London

Boyd H 1981 Introduction to homoeopathic medicine. Beaconsfield, Beaconsfield

Day C 1988 Clinical trials in bovine mastitis. British Homoeopathic Journal 75: 11–14

Faculty of Homoeopathy 1993 Non-medically qualified practitioners of homoeopathy. British Homoeopathic Journal with Simile 82

Haehl R 1985 Samuel Hahnemann. His life and work. B Jain, New Delhi, India, 2 vols

Koehler G 1986 Handbook of homoeopathy. Thorsons, London

Livingston R 1991 Homoeopathy evergreen medicine. Jewel in the medical crown. Asher Asher, Poole

Tyler-Kent J 1979 Lectures in homoeopathic philosophy. Thorsons, Wellingborough

FURTHER READING – JOURNALS

Engineer S J, Vakil A E, Engineer L S 1990 A study of antibody formation by Baptisia tinctoria O in experimental animals. British Homoeopathic Journal 79: 109–113

Fox A D 1993 General practice management of gastrointestinal problems assisted by Vegatest techniques. British Homoeopathic Journal 82: 87–91

Gaucher C, Jeulin D, Peycru P, Pla A, Amengual C 1993 Cholera and homoeopathic medicine. British Homoeopathic Journal 82: 155–163

Jacobs J, Jiminez L M, Gloyd S, Caraes F E, Gaitan M P, Crowthers D 1993 Homoeopathic treatment of acute childhood diarrhoea. British Homoeopathic Journal 82: 83–86

Linde W, Melchart D, Jonas W B, Hornung J 1994 Ways to enhance the quality and acceptance of clinical and laboratory studies in homoeopathy. British Homoeopathic Journal 83: 3–7

Mokkapatti R 1992 An experimental double-blind study to evaluate the use of Euphrasia in preventing conjunctivitis. British Homoeopathic Journal 81: 22–24

Rastogi D P, Singh V P, Singh V, Dey S K 1993 Evaluation of homoeopathic therapy in 129 asymptomatic HIV carriers. British Homoeopathic Journal 82: 4–8

Vozianov A F, Simeonova N K 1990 Homoeopathic treatment of patients with adenomas of the prostate. British Homoeopathic Journal 79: 148–151

FURTHER READING – BOOKS

Blackie M 1986 Classical homoeopathy. Beaconsfield, Beaconsfield

Boyd H 1981 Introduction to homoeopathic medicine. Beaconsfield, Beaconsfield

Hubbard E W 1990 Homoeopathy as art and science. Beaconsfield, Beaconsfield

Livingston R 1991 Homoeopathy evergreen medicine. The jewel in the medical crown. Asher Asher, Poole

Lockie A 1989 The family guide to homoeopathy. Hamish Hamilton, London
Resch G, Gutmann V 1987 Scientific foundations of homoeopathy. Barthel and Barthel, St Ottillien, Germany
Smith T 1986 Talking about homoeopathy. Insight, Worthing
Tyler-Kent J 1979 Lectures in homoeopathic philosophy. Thorsons, Wellingborough.

USEFUL ADDRESSES

Any professional nurse interested in training in homoeopathy should ensure that the course is nationally accredited and has statutory recognition. It is helpful to obtain a copy of the Faculty of Homoeopathy Statement entitled 'Non-medically qualified practitioners of homoeopathy' referred to in the Reference list.

Dr M Money
Course Administrator
Trueman Building
Liverpool John Moores University
15/21 Webster Street
Liverpool L3 2ET

Accredited MSc (Homoeopathic Medicine) degree programme. Registered nurse applicants may complete the first module to certificate level.

Faculty of Homoeopathy
Royal London Homoeopathic Hospital
Gt Ormond Street
London WC1N 3HR

Accredited courses for registered nurses, midwives and pharmacists.

Faculty of Homoeopathy
Glasgow Homoeopathic Hospital
100 Great Western Road
Glasgow G12 ONR

Accredited courses for registered nurses, midwives and pharmacists.

Centre for Complementary Medicine (North West)
Stockport College of Further & Higher Education
Wellington Road South
Stockport SK1 3UQ

For further details contact Denise Rankin-Box, Senior Lecturer in Nursing & Health Studies. Discussions underway to establish accredited modular courses for health care professionals.

Institute of Complementary Medicine
PO Box 194
London SE16 1QZ

Discussions underway to establish accredited courses for registered nurses and health professionals.

Centre For the Study of Complementary Medicine
51 Bedford Place
Southampton
Hampshire S01 2DG

The Centre offers post-graduate courses in the scientific evaluation of homoeopathic therapy to medical doctors, dentists and registered nurses. Applicants should have a background in homoeopathic medicine. The Centre has carried out much of the leading scientific research in homoeopathic and complementary therapies and publishes its findings on a regular basis.

14 Humour and laughter therapy

Jane Mallett

Humour and laughter therapy — *amusing intervention used by the health care professional or patient to produce a beneficial response in the patient.*

Humour can be viewed from physical, psychological and sociological perspectives and is difficult to define. A simplistic definition of a humorous comment is: communication (verbal and non-verbal) intended to cause amusement. However, humour can be used for different reasons including reducing the patient's anxiety (Robinson 1977, Mallett 1993), relief of hostility and aggression (Robinson 1977) and discussion of taboo topics (Emerson 1969). Recent research by the author has shown that humour between nurses and patients may be used to maintain 'friendly reciprocity' when discussing potentially contentious issues (Mallett 1994a).

Humour would seem to be more than simply producing talk or gestures intended to cause amusement and it is used for a number of reasons in natural conversations between the nurse and patient. Thus, it should be considered within the context in which it is produced.

Research on communication between health care professionals and patients in hospital has also indicated that humour and laughter are used naturally, for instance, to convey feelings such as anxiety, fear, anger, embarrassment, etc. in an indirect fashion (Robinson 1977). This could potentially be of use in therapy but should only be used following proper evaluation of the intervention.

The science of laughter is known as gelotology. This refers to the stimulus of humour with subsequent emotional and behavioural responses (Fry 1986). Laughter is generally taken to be the physical expression of humour (Keith-Spiegel 1972). Once again, this definition requires further qualification since laughter is also socially managed and organized in conversation (Jefferson 1979).

In addition, there are some reported instances of inappropriate laughter as a consequence of poisoning (for example with ethyl alcohol) or disease (Moody 1978, Goldstein 1982). An illustration of the latter is the Fore tribe of New Guinea who suffer from 'Kuru' or 'laughing death'. Caused by a virus, the disease is spread by the ritual ingestion of brain tissue. The terminal stage is apparently marked by uncontrolled, hilarious and uproarious laughter (Gajdusek & Zigas 1959).

There are also cultural, sex and age differences in the use of humour and laughter. For instance, eskimos have been reported to use humour to resolve quarrels — whoever gains most laughter from the audience while insulting their opponents wins the argument (Robinson 1977). In 1978, Adams & Kirkevold studied people in a restaurant and reported differences in the amount of laughter according to age and sex. Overall, females laughed and smiled more than males but amongst females the 12–17 age group laughed most compared with the greatest frequency of laughter in the 18–22 age group of males. The research highlights that gender and age differences need to be taken into account when considering the use of humour and laughter as tools for therapy.

Further specific effects or uses of humour and laughter have been investigated in the fields of physiology, psychology and sociology. The clinical significance of this research is not yet clear but may turn out to have important implications for health care.

The physical responses to humour and laughter affect most of the major systems of our bodies (Fry 1986). These include an increase in heart rate, blood pressure and muscle tension which is followed by a decrease (Berlyne 1972, Chapman 1976, Fry 1986, Fry & Savin 1988). In addition, salivary immunoglobulin A (IgA) concentration and spontaneous lymphocyte blastogenesis have been found to increase, and adrenalin and cortisol secretion to decrease, following viewing of a humorous video by healthy adults (Dillon et al 1985, Berk et al 1988a,b).

Psychological research has shown that humour can have a part in reducing anxiety. A study by Nemeth (1979) indicated that people who watched a humorous film had significantly decreased anxiety levels compared with those who watched a non-humorous film.

Sick joke cycles (e.g. following the Chernobyl disaster — 'What has feathers and glows in the dark? Chicken Kiev') have been studied from a sociological perspective (Dundes 1987). It is suggested that these act as a collective mental defence mechanism to allow people to articulate and cope with the worst disasters (Dundes 1987).

The results of these inquiries may prove useful to nurses caring for patients. Humour and laughter (and their use and effects) are not always clearly differentiated in the literature and in reality, it may not be possible to separate the two. Also, much of the research on humour or laughter originates in the United States, is conducted on healthy adults and is non-clinical. Since the use of humour and laughter is related to culture, and patients have physical, psychological, social and spiritual problems that healthy adults may not have, care must be taken when using the findings and recommendations of the research in health care environments within the UK (Mallett 1994b).

HISTORICAL BACKGROUND

The benefits of humour and laughter have long been recognized and are mentioned in the bible; Proverbs 17:22 states 'A cheerful heart does good like a medicine: but a broken spirit makes one sick' (Living Bible 1971). More recently it has been suggested that humour and/or laughter may be used therapeutically in a number of ways (Moody 1978, Goldstein 1982):

- to aid recovery from surgery (Henri de Mondeville, 13th-century surgeon)
- as a cure for melancholy (Robert Burton, 16th-century English parson and scholar)
- as physical exercise (Richard Mulcaster, 16th-century physician)
- as a way to release excess tension (Herbert Spencer, 17th-century sociologist)
- to restore equilibrium (Immanuel Kant, 18th-century German philosopher)
- to use in treatment of the sick (William Battie, 18th-century English physician)
- to help digestion (Gottlieb Hufeland, 19th-century German professor)
- to stimulate the internal organs (James Walsh, 20th-century American physician).

One of the most influential proponents of humour and laughter therapy of modern times who has probably been responsible for the upsurge in interest since the 1970s, is Norman Cousins. His documented experiences as a patient and subsequent writings on the value of humour and laughter in health care (Cousins 1976, 1979, 1989) have done much to stimulate the imagination of professionals. This appears true, particularly in the USA where these types of therapies are currently popular and seem to have encouraged much supportive business (for example, the Humor Project).

TREATMENT

Humour or laughter therapy may take the form of making funny pictures to decorate the patient's room, sending singing telegrams, showing home or humorous movies, using puppets to increase playfulness and clowns to facilitate communication and responsiveness (Cousins 1976, Moody 1978, Simon 1989, Erdman 1991).

Literature describing humour or laughter 'therapy' in clinical practice is sparse, although Erdman (1991) relates the setting up of a 'Laugh Mobile' which was wheeled round to patients in their rooms twice a week. Examples of items on the Laugh Mobile included: Play Doh (a soft modelling clay), colouring books, finger paint, Mr Bubble® (a pipe for blowing bubbles), water guns, humorous books, videotapes and audiotapes, games and puzzles. Erdman (1991) describes the 'success' of the therapy and illustrates this with examples of how patients reacted:

'A 42-year-old patient with lymphoma was the first patient to select Mr Bubble from the humour cart. He laughed like a child as he blew sparkly bubbles that burst when they touched his smiling visitors' (p. 1362).

Before introducing an intervention, careful assessment of the patient is necessary to ensure that humour therapy is appropriate (Simon 1989, Erdman 1991). Three criteria are useful for determining whether or not humour will be helpful. These are:

- timing — for example, humour could be considered unacceptable at the height of a crisis
- receptiveness — what might be funny to a patient at one time might not be humorous at another
- content — ensure that the patient does not feel that the humour is happening at his/her expense (Burton Leiber 1986).

Patients also initiate their own humour and laughter therapy to help them overcome the awfulness of their situation. Bruning (1985), who discovered that she had breast cancer at the age of 31 and underwent chemotherapy, wrote how she sometimes 'spent more time joking and laughing than being treated', while Cousins (1976), who suffered from ankylosing spondylitis, watched Candid Camera films and found that 10 minutes of genuine belly laughter had an anaesthetic effect that would give him 2 hours of pain-free sleep.

Therapeutic potential in nursing

Although some research exists which provides evidence that humour may be an effective intervention this is not robust (Hunt 1993). Since little formal, systematic and rigorous evaluation of humour and laughter as tools for clinical therapy has been conducted, the therapeutic benefits of humour and laughter remain unproven (Mallett 1994b). Some possible benefits are as follows:

- To facilitate patient teaching and improve recall
- To reduce anxiety
- To assist communication (including with psychiatric patients)
- To enhance feelings of well-being
- To positively influence hopefulness
- To aid speech therapy
- To act as an 'icebreaker'
- To reduce pain.

See also Cousins 1076, Moody 1970, Potter & Goodman 1983, Hinds et al 1984, Napora 1985, Parfitt 1990, Gaberson 1991, Hunt 1993.

In addition, a number of studies on healthy adults indicate that humour and laughter have specific effects which may be of benefit in, for example:

- Enhancing the immune system (Dillon et al 1985, Berk et al 1988a,b)
- Increasing discomfort thresholds (Cogan et al 1987)
- Reducing muscle tension (Fry 1986)
- Assisting with cardiac and respiratory therapy (Fry 1986)
- 'Stress-buffering' (Martin & Lefcourt 1983) and coping (Coombs & Goldman 1973).

These effects may be useful within the clinical field but research is necessary with patients to evaluate their use in practice.

Contraindications for use

Opinions differ on which types of humour may not be appropriate in therapy. This may be because there is a lack of agreement on what constitutes negative humour (Mallett 1994b). Generally, contraindications are considered in terms of what humour is used to achieve.

- Humour is destructive if used to mask hostility, ridicule or 'put down' the recipient.

- Humour is inappropriate in the midst of a crisis or when it ignores the patients' humour 'styles' (Burton Leiber 1986, Hunt 1993).

- Sexist, sexual, racial and self-deprecating humour should be avoided (Burton Leiber 1986, Hunt 1993, Simon 1989); however, this may be part of the patient's style and difficult to preclude.

- Understanding the patient's cultural background and sexuality is important in avoiding non-therapeutic humour. For example, in Spanish-American people illness is regarded as a form of punishment and joking may be taken seriously if it indicates blame (Robinson 1977).

- Recognition of male patients' use of humour to assert their masculinity to female nurses (Robinson 1977) can prevent inappropriate responses to their teasing.

The use (and the nature, purpose and understanding) of humour depends on the situation and context in which it is produced (Mallett 1994b) and there may be few contraindications that apply absolutely in all situations.

Summary

There is much anecdotal 'evidence' from nurses and patients to support humour and laughter as therapy. However, there is little research to support specific humour or laughter interventions as beneficial in the short or long term in the clinical environment. Humour and laughter remain potentially exciting and innovative tools for nursing therapy. They have a number of effects which could prove beneficial for many different nursing and medical diagnoses and appear to have the additional advantage of being adaptable to most situations. More clinical evaluation of humour and laughter therapy is required before its appropriate use can be defined.

REFERENCES

Adams R M, Kirkevold B 1978 Looking, smiling, laughing and moving in restaurants: sex and age differences. Environmental Psychology and Non-Verbal Behaviour 3: 117–121

Berk L S, Tan S A, Nehlsen-Cannarella S L, Napier B J, Lee J W, Lewis J E, Hubbard R W, Eby W C, Fry W F 1988a Mirth modulates adrenocorticomedullary activity: suppression of cortisol and epinephrine. Clinical Research 36: 121A

Berk L S, Tan S A, Nehlsen-Cannarella S L, Napier B J, Lewis J E, Lee J W, Eby W C, Fry W F 1988b Humor associated laughter decreases cortisol and increases spontaneous lymphocyte blastogenesis. Clinical Research 36: 435A

Berlyne D E 1972 Humor and its kin. In: Goldstein J H, McGhee P E (eds) The psychology of humor. Academic Press, London, p 43–60

Bruning N 1985 Coping with chemotherapy. Dial Press, Doubleday, New York

Burton Leiber D 1986 Laughter and humor in critical care. Dimensions of Critical Care Nursing 5: 102–170

Chapman A J 1976 Social aspects of humorous laughter. In: Chapman A J, Foot H C (eds) Humor and laughter: theory, research and applications. John Wiley, London, p 155–185

Cogan R, Cogan D, Waltz W, McCue M 1987 Effects of laughter and relaxation on discomfort thresholds. Journal of Behavioral Medicine. 10: 139–144

Coombs R H, Goldman L J 1973 Maintenance and discontinuity of coping mechanisms in an intensive care unit. Social Problems 20: 342–355

Cousins N 1976 Anatomy of an illness (as perceived by the patient). New England Journal of Medicine 295: 1458–1463

Cousins N 1979 Anatomy of an illness. Bantam, New York

Cousins N 1989 Head first the biology of hope. EP Dutton, New York

Dillon K M, Minchoff B, Baker K H 1985 Positive emotional states and enhancement of the immune system. International Journal of Psychiatry in Medicine 15: 13–18

Dundes A 1987 At ease, disease-AIDS jokes as sick humor. American Behavioral Scientist 30: 72–81

Emerson J P 1969 Negotiating the serious import of humor. Sociometry (Journal of Research in Social Psychology) 32: 169–181

Erdman L 1991 Laughter therapy for patients with cancer. Oncology Nursing Forum 18: 1359–1363

Fry W F 1986 Humor, physiology, and the aging process. In: Nahemow L, McCluskey-Fawcett K A, McGhee P E (eds) Humor and aging. Academic Press, London, p 81–98

Fry W F, Savin W M 1988 Mirthful laughter and blood pressure. Humor — International Journal of Humor Research 1: 49–62

Gaberson K B 1991 The effect of humorous distraction on preoperative anxiety. AORN 54: 1258–1263 (cited in Hunt 1993)

Gajdusek D C, Zigas V 1978 Kuru. American Journal of Medicine 26: 442 (cited in Moody 1978)

Goldstein J H 1982 Laugh a day, can mirth keep disease at bay? Sciences 22: 21–25

Hinds P S, Martin J, Vogel R J 1984 Nursing strategies to influence adolescent hopefulness during oncologic illness. Journal of Pediatric Oncology Nursing 4: 14–22 (cited in Hunt 1993)

Hunt A H 1993 Humor as a nursing intervention. Cancer Nursing 16: 34–39

Keith-Spiegel P 1972 Early conceptions of humor: varieties and issues. In: Goldstein J H, McGhee P E (eds) The psychology of humor. Academic Press, London, p 3–39

Jefferson G 1979 A technique for inviting laughter and its subsequent acceptance or declination. In: Psathas G (ed) Everyday language studies in ethnomethodology. Irvington, New York, p 79–95

Living Bible 1971 Tyndale House, UK

Mallett J 1993 Use of humour and laughter in patient care. British Journal of Nursing 2: 172–175

Mallett J 1994a Unpublished research

Mallett J 1994b Humour therapy. In: Wells R, Tschudin V (eds) Wells' supportive therapies in health care. Baillière Tindall, London, p 214–238

Martin R A, Lefcourt H M 1983 Sense of humor as a moderator of the relation between stressors and moods. Journal of Personality and Social Psychology 45: 1313–1324

Moody R A 1978 Laugh after laugh, the healing power of humor. Headwaters, Florida

Napora J 1985 A study of the effects of a program of humorous activity on the subjective well-being of senior adults. Dissertation Abstracts International 46: 276–A

Nemeth P 1979 An investigation into the relationship between humor and anxiety. Dissertation Abstracts International 40: 1378–B

Parfitt J M 1990 Humorous preoperative teaching. AORN 52: 114–120 (cited in Hunt 1993)

Potter R E, Goodman N J 1983 The implementation of laughter as a therapy facilitator with adult aphasics. Journal of Communication Disorders 16: 41–48

Robinson V 1977 Humor in nursing. In: Carlson C E, Blackwell B 1977 Behavioural concepts and nursing intervention, 2nd edn. JP Lippincott, USA, p 191–210

Simon J 1989 Humor techniques for oncology nurses. Oncology Nursing Forum 16: 667–670

KEY REFERENCES

Coser R L 1959 Some social functions of laughter, a study of humor in a hospital setting. Human Relations XII: 171–182
One of the first and most important pieces of sociological humour research within a hospital environment. Uses patients' jocular talk to illustrate how

humour is used, for example, to ward off danger, as a means of rebellion against authority, and as a relief from mechanical routine.

Fox Tennant K 1986 The effect of humor on the recovery rate of cataract
    patients: a pilot study. In: Nahemow L, McCluskey-Fawcett K A, McGhee
    P E (eds) Humor and aging. Academic Press, London, p 245–251
This chapter details a small study of 20 patients to determine the effect of humour on the recovery rate of elderly patients after cataract surgery. While the study does not identify any significant findings it does illustrate the kind of research that may be useful in clarifying more precisely the role of humour in health care.

Schmitt N 1990 Patients' perception of laughter in a rehabilitation hospital.
    Rehabilitation Nursing 15: 143–146
This paper provides the results of a small survey conducted on 35 patients in a rehabilitation hospital. The questionnaire included items with which patients were requested to indicate strong agreement to strong disagreement on a five-point scale. The data showed that patients welcome laughter and perceive nurses who laugh with them to be therapeutic.

Simon J M 1988 Humour and the older adult: implications for nursing.
    Journal of Advanced Nursing 13: 441–446
This is a correlational descriptive study of 24 adults over 61 years old from a senior citizen community centre in Texas. The research examined the relationship between the uses of humour and health outcomes as measured by perceived health, life satisfaction and morale in older adults. The findings demonstrated significant positive relationships between situational humour and perceived health and situational humour and morale, and a negative relationship between coping humour and perceived health.

USEFUL ADDRESSES

American Association for
Therapeutic Humor
1163 Shermer Road,
Northbrook
Illinois 60062–4538, USA

Humor Project
110 Spring Street
Saratoga Springs
NY 12866, USA

International Society for Humor
Studies
c/o Don LF Nilsen
English Department
Arizona State University

Tempe
Arizona 85287–0302, USA
Tel: 602 965 7592, Fax: 602 965 3451

Journal of Nursing Jocularity
PO Box 40416
Mesa
Arizona 85274, USA
Tel: 602 835 6165

Laughter Clinic
Robert W Holden
34 Denewood Avenue
Handsworth Wood
Birmingham B20 2AB
Tel: 0121 551 2932

15 Hypnosis

Denise Rankin-Box

Hypnosis — *the deliberate use of a trance state to enhance the sense of health and well-being.*

Trance is commonly described as an altered state of consciousness, rather like day-dreaming, when the brain appears to 'switch off' for a few seconds. This natural state may occur several times each day; however, conscious use of the trance state can help in self-healing.

Induced trance states have been used throughout the centuries and across a range of cultures and continents such as India, China and Egypt (Conachy 1994) and North America, Africa, Greece and Britain (Booth 1993). The trance state described, commonly resulted from a rhythmical, repetitive activity such as swaying or dancing, as well as auditory or visual cues.

Hypnosis is the conscious use of the natural trance state and seems to provide a link with the unconscious mind through suggestion. Suggestion refers to the presentation of an idea to a client, and the extent to which the client accepts the idea (suggestibility) is influenced by motivation and expectation. There is no definitive research to adequately explain this phemonenon. Despite this, whilst suggestion promotes a largely psychological or placebo-like response, it is possible to anaesthetize parts of the body and influence the autonomic nervous system which is not usually under voluntary control (Whorwell et al 1992, Chakraverty et al 1992).

Contrary to popular belief, the therapist does not take control of the client. In effect, all hypnosis is self-hypnosis (Vickers 1993). The therapist acts only as a facilitator and can help an individual to work towards an improvement in their health and well-being. Hypnotherapy is primarily a self-care technique and could be used, for example, in stress management, chronic and acute pain control, and management of pain during labour and dental surgery. Hypnosis can also help in resolving stammers, phobias, facial ticks and habits such as smoking or overeating. However, it is important to appreciate that the client must *want* to solve his/her problem.

HISTORICAL BACKGROUND

Western recognition of hypnosis was initiated by Franz Mesmer (1734–1815) in 1773. He believed that some form of fluid could be redistributed by the force of magnetic poles. Although experiencing considerable popularity for a while, the scientific basis of this 'animal magnetism' was largely discredited and Mesmer denounced. Interest in Mesmerism was revived again in the nineteenth century, most notably by James Braid who used the term 'hypnosis'. Braid suggested that Mesmer's clients had been in a trance state which could be induced in a number of ways such as watching a swinging pendulum or staring at a distant point or light (Booth 1993). Braid called this 'neurohypnotism' from the Greek *hypnos* meaning sleep since he thought that the trance state induced a neurological response similar to but different from sleep.

During World War 1, Simmel developed a technique called 'hypnoanalysis' for treating war neurosis (Tamin 1988). More recent developments in this field are described by Erickson & Rossi (1980) and Spiegel & Spiegel (1978). Hypnotism is gaining popularity in health care and has been recommended for study by the British and American Medical Associations (Booth 1993).

TREATMENT

Initially the therapist takes a general history from the client and identifies problems of current concern. Trance induction can take many forms and therapists may choose a technique to suit the client. Commonly, subjects are asked to focus on a point and let their breathing become slow and regular. As their eyelids become heavy, they are asked to close them and start to relax. The clients control the extent to which they relax into the trance state.

Guided visualization techniques such as imagining a walk along a beach or in a garden are practised with caution since they may not always trigger a positive response; for example, strong images of summer days have been known to initiate asthma attacks and an imaginary tour around a house could induce claustrophobia. It may be preferable to ask the client to imagine a scene or a place in which they would feel contented and relaxed.

A therapist ends the trance state gradually, allowing the client to control the speed at which he emerges from the trance state. Reorientation may be facilitated by the therapist counting back from three to one.

Descriptions of the trance state vary from an altered state of consciousness similar to a meditative state to a heightened sense of awareness. It is not uncommon for individuals to feel very relaxed or have sensations of heaviness or lightness. The hypnotherapist's voice may fade away as the client becomes more relaxed.

Stages of technique

Induction — commonly linked to a relaxation technique.

Trigger — may be used to enable deeper relaxed states to occur by suggestion.

Deepening (ideo-motor response) — refers to client's response to questions using, for example, finger movement rather than a spoken reply, to facilitate deeper relaxation.

Therapy — the stage where the client's concerns are addressed, e.g. becoming less anxious, more assertive, ego-boosting.

Lightener/reorientation — the client is gently reorientated with his surroundings before coming out of the trance state.

Ending — the client is reorientated and commonly it is suggested that he will come out of trance after counting from 3 to 1.

Therapeutic potential in nursing

Some examples of potential applications of hypnosis in nursing practice are as follows:

- Relaxation
- Acute and chronic pain management
- Childbirth — management of labour pain
- Stress management
- Control of certain phobias — needle phobia during, for example, renal dialysis, chemotherapy, diabetes
- Post-amputation phantom pain management
- Relief of nausea during pregnancy, drug treatment or post-operatively
- In casualty simple trance techniques may be used to relax or 'numb' an area requiring suturing — this can be effective in both children and adults

- Insomnia
- Hypertension
- Irritable bowel syndrome
- Self-hypnosis — taught to clients for pain control in labour, acute anxiety attacks, insomnia, relaxation and so on.

Contraindications for use

- Whilst hypnosis can be extremely valuable it is important that the therapist is competent to deal with the particular problem.
- Avoid long-standing psychological problems which may require professional counselling/treatment.
- Occasionally clients may feel lightheaded when coming out of a deep trance state and it important to know how to manage this and any abreactions that may occur.

Summary

Hypnosis has considerable potential for use within nursing practice. The possible applications are wide-ranging and it is a therapy which gives clients responsibility for their own healing. Whether it can be used effectively in the clinical setting depends largely on the clients' willingness to manage their own health care; the therapist acts only as a facilitator of the healing process.

REFERENCES

Booth B 1993 Complementary therapy. Nursing Times/Macmillan, London

Chakraverty K et al 1992 Erythromyalgia: the role of hypnotherapy. Postgraduate Medical Journal 68: 44–46

Conachy S 1994 Hypnotherapy. In: Wells R, Tschudin V (eds) Wells' supportive therapies in health care. Baillière Tindall, London

Erickson M, Rossi E 1980 (eds) Innovative hypnotherapy – the collected papers of Milton H. Erickson on hypnosis. Irvington, New York, vol IV

Spiegel H, Spiegel D 1978 Trance and treatment: clinical uses of hypnosis. Basic Books, New York

Tamin J 1988 Hypnosis. In: Rankin-Box D F (ed) Complementary health therapies: a guide for nurses and the caring professions. Croom Helm, Beckenham, Kent, pp 189–202

Vickers A 1993 Complementary medicine and disability: alternatives for people with disabling conditions. Chapman and Hall, London
Whorwell P J et al 1992 Physiological effects of emotion: assessment via hypnosis. Lancet 340: 69–72

FURTHER READING – JOURNALS

Chakraverty K et al 1992 Erythromyalgia: the role of hypnotherapy. Postgraduate Medical Journal 68: 44–46
Chapman L F, Goodell H, Wolff H G 1959 Changes in tissue vulnerability induced during hypnotic suggestion. Journal of Psychosomatic Research 4: 99–105
Contach P, Hockenbury M, Herman S 1985 Self-hypnosis as antiemetic therapy in children receiving chemotherapy. Oncology Nursing Forum 12: 41–46
Ewer T C, Stewart D E 1986 Improvement of bronchial hyperresponsiveness in patients with moderate asthma after treatment with a hypnotic technique: a randomised controlled trial. British Journal of Medicine (Clinical Research) 293: 1129–1132
Holroyd J, Hill A 1989 Pushing the limits of recovery: hypnotherapy with a stroke patient. International Journal of Clinical and Experimental Hypnosis 37: 120–128
Maslach C, Marshall G, Zimbardo P G 1972 Hypnotic control of peripheral skin temperature: a case report. Psychophysiology 9: 600–605
Minichello W E 1987 Treatment of hyperhidrosis of amputation site with hypnosis and suggestions involving classical conditioning. International Journal of Psychosomatics 34: 7–8
Negley-Parker E, Araoz D L 1986 Hypnotherapy with families of chronically ill children. International Journal of Psychosomatics 33: 9–11
Whorwell P J et al 1992 Physiological effects of emotion: assessment via hypnosis. Lancet 340: 69–72

FURTHER READING – BOOKS

Bandler R 1985 Using your brain for a change. Real People Press, Utah
Garner G, Olness K (eds) 1981 Hypnosis and hypnotherapy with children. Grune & Stratton, New York
Hartland J 1971 Medical and dental hypnosis. Baillière Tindall, London
Rosen S (ed) 1982 My voice will go with you: the teaching tales of Milton Erickson. WW Norton, London
Spiegel H, Spiegel D 1978 Trance and treatment: clinical uses of hypnosis. Basic Books, New York
Young P 1987 Personal change through self-hypnosis. Angus and Robertson, London

USEFUL ADDRESSES

At present there are no nationally accredited courses in hypnosis. The Institute of Complementary Medicine maintains a register of hypnotherapists affiliated to professional organizations.

British Hypnosis Research
Southpoint
8 Paston Place
Brighton BN2 1HA
Tel: 01273 693622

British Hypnotherapy Association
1 Wythburn Place
London W1H 5Wl
Tel: 0171 262 8852/723 4443

British Society of Medical and
Dental Hypnosis
48 Links Road
Ashtead
Surrey KT31 3JH
Tel: 01372 273522

National College for Hypnotherapy
and Psychotherapy
12 Cross Street
Nelson
Lancs

Owl College of Hypnosis
2 Buchanan Street
Leigh
Greater Manchester WN7 1XT

Therapy Training College
8–10 Balaclava Street
Kings Heath
Birmingham B14 7SG
Tel: 0121 444 5435

UK Training College of
Hypnotherapy and Counselling
10 Alexander Street
London W2 5NT
Tel: 0171 221 1796/727 2006

World Federation of
Hypnotherapists
Belmont Square
46 Belmont Road
Ramsgate
Kent CT11 7QG
Tel: 01843 587929

16 Massage

Carol Horrigan

Massage — *a conscious, deliberate, and often formalized use of the instinctive response to comfort another person using touch.*

The many systems of massage practised now in the UK have all been adopted from other cultures. They can be stimulating or sedating, vigorous or gentle and include all or part of the patient's body; they may be performed using the practitioner's hands, feet, elbows or knees as well as instruments or machines. Some methods use oil, cream or a lotion to lubricate the skin; for others, talcum powder is preferred. The patient lies on a couch or bed, although some therapists prefer to work on a thin mattress or rug on the floor. Massage does not have to include the whole body or take more than an hour to complete. Apart from this being impractical for a nurse massage therapist, many patients are too unwell to tolerate more than 10–20 minutes of massage and this is usually sufficient to achieve the desired effect. Massage can usually be adapted to the circumstances.

British people have a reputation for being reserved and touch or caress is considered a private and intimate activity, often linked with sex. The increase in foreign travel and contact with immigrants from other cultures have helped to create a more relaxed society in which physical expressions of gratitude or affection are becoming acceptable. In this climate, massage as a therapeutic intervention is more likely to gain recognition.

Many claims are made for the effects of massage. Some of these have been investigated and upheld by research, for example, Acolet et al (1993) regarding physiological changes; other claims are in contention (Barr & Taslitz 1970, Reed & Held 1988, Ferrel-Torry & Glick 1993); but many remain anecdotal and need substantiation.

HISTORICAL BACKGROUND

The word massage derives from Arabic, Greek, Hindi and French words associated with touch, pressing or shampooing. Both the Bible and the Koran refer to anointing the skin with oil (Beck 1988). Documents (in the British Museum) describe massage being performed around 3000 BC in China. Various techniques were refined by the Japanese and Middle Eastern cultures as part of their health and hygiene routines. The Greeks and Romans used massage to prepare soldiers and gladiators. However, in the Middle Ages religious dogma and superstition regarded anything related to physical or emotional pleasure as sinful. Not until the Renaissance did a renewed interest in aesthetics and health reinstate massage as a beneficial activity.

In 1870, massage was introduced to the United States from Europe, and in 1884 the first book on the subject was published there. That same year, a group of women in England formed the Society of Trained Masseuses which later became the Chartered Society of Physiotherapists (1964). During both World Wars massage was used in the rehabilitation of injured men. Archives at the University College and Middlesex Schools of Nursing show that nurses were being trained in massage in the early twentieth century. However, the increased use of technology led to a decline in the use of massage by both nurses and physiotherapists. There has been a gradual resurgence of massage in nursing since the 1970s. Beginning in the care of the elderly and care of the dying, it is gaining recognition now in all nursing specialties.

TREATMENT

Massage, like any other intervention, needs to be planned following an assessment of the patient and evaluated when it has been implemented. Preparations for massage should include the following:

- Identifying the problems that massage may be able to relieve
- Ascertaining positions that the patient may or may not be able to adopt
- Checking that all medications/interventions are completed for the period of the massage
- Making sure the patient is comfortable (bladder, bowels, respiratory function, pain control)
- Ensuring the massage will be undisturbed (single room, 'do not disturb' sign)
- Having adequate facilities (heating, towels, pillows, adjustable bed, comfortable chair)

- Explaining the rationale for massage to the patient/relatives and proceeding only if they agree to it (Baldwin 1986, De Wever 1977).

The rhythmic movement of massage is comforting and relaxing, and the patient will want to rest afterwards. Lifting equipment or colleagues to help with any transfer should be arranged before the massage to avoid disrupting its relaxing effects.

The therapist will adjust every massage session to suit the patient's needs, desires and tolerance, but some measures and processes are almost always included:

- The therapist prepares (in her preferred way) to ensure a calm frame of mind; all other responsibilities are accounted for, and an assessment of the patient is made.

- The working area is prepared with adequate heating, 'do not disturb' signs, towels, blankets, pillows and massage oil.

- The patient is made comfortable and covered with towels to expose only the part of the body being massaged, so that dignity and warmth are maintained at all times.

- Massage begins and ends with slow, stroking movements (effleurage); this ensures a sense of calm and relaxation.

- A range of massage movements and gentle passive exercise of the muscles or joints is carried out in a logical order, according to the style of massage being used.

- Finally, the patient is warmly covered, the therapist indicates that treatment is completed and the patient is left to rest.

Therapeutic potential in nursing

Research has indicated that massage can have the following beneficial effects:

- Reduction in anxiety levels (Acolet 1993, Field et al 1993, Fraser & Ross Kerr 1993)
- Emotional stress relief (Longworth 1982, Mckecknie 1983)
- Relief of muscular tension and fatigue (Balke et al 1989)
- Improved local and distant lymphatic circulation (Morgan et al 1992, Mortimer 1990)
- Better local blood circulation, leading to a feeling of warmth (Hovind & Neilsen 1974, Kaada & Torsteinbo 1989)
- Pain relief due to the release of endorphins, leading to relaxation (Kaada & Torsteinbo 1989).

Contraindications for use

- Extremes of body temperature
  - if a patient is hypothermic, massage may increase surface circulation and seriously reduce core temperature
  - the same mechanism would exacerbate the discomfort of the patient with pyrexia who also may not wish to be touched
- Contagious diseases/acute infections
  - besides disturbing body temperature, there is the danger of disease transmission
- Acute, undiagnosed back pain
  - this may be simple muscular spasm or potentially dangerous compression of the spinal cord; no massage should be carried out until a diagnosis has been made
- Fractures
  - massage cannot be carried out directly over fracture sites but it is useful, when applied to other areas of the body, for relaxing orthopaedic patients
- Cardiovascular instability (hypertension, angina, cardiac oedema)
  - massage is beneficial only if given in short, non-tiring sessions
- Respiratory insufficiency
  - patients may need to remain sitting upright during massage and this can be arranged
- Deep vein thrombosis — *never massage feet, legs or trunk*
  - very light hand or face massage will not increase circulation enough to move emboli, and may reduce patient's anxiety
- Varicose veins/phlebitis
  - massage here requires a specialized technique, not taught by most massage schools. Standard pressures and movements may induce itching, causing the patient to scratch and accidentally damage the veins
- Low platelet count and other causes of easy bruising
  - this includes patients with leukaemia, purpura, and those receiving chemotherapy, radiotherapy, or high-dose anticoagulant therapy
  - provided the massage is very gentle and care is taken when massaging over bony prominences, the patient will benefit
- Unexplained lumps and bumps
  - these should be diagnosed before massage
- Unstable pregnancy
  - Massage should not be given to the abdomen, legs and feet for the first trimester
- Cancer patients
  - metastases are not caused or spread by gentle surface massage (McNamara 1993)

- chemotherapy and radiotherapy may make the skin very dry
- some radiologists will not permit massage to areas currently undergoing radiotherapy
- lymphoedema requires a special type of massage and should not be attempted by the untrained
- Chronic fatigue syndrome
  - patients can usually only tolerate short treatments when the syndrome is active
- People with HIV/AIDS
  - many of the conditions above will apply
  - loss of weight and/or Karposi's sarcoma may make massage uncomfortable unless a gentle touch and extra lubricant are used
- Dermatology patients
  - very few skin diseases are contagious, but infection is a risk if the patient has broken skin
- Rheumatoid arthritis and osteoarthrosis
  - careful positioning of the patient and frequent change of position may be required
- Dementia and psychosis
  - such patients may be confused or frightened by massage and its effects
- Contact lenses
  - some types should not be worn with the eyes shut; check that the patient has removed them.

Summary

Massage can be used in nursing in the form of gentle application of hand lotion or with advanced techniques for symptom control. For the patient it is a welcome contrast to the technological procedures of modern medicine.

Touch is an integral aspect of communication and nursing care where the use of massage can promote a relaxing and therapeutic environment.

REFERENCES

Acolet D et al 1993 Changes in plasma cortisol and catecholamine concentrations in response to massage in pre-term infants. Archives of Disease in Childhood 68: 29–31

Baldwin L C 1986 The therapeutic use of touch with the elderly. Physical and Occupational Therapy in Geriatrics 4: 45–50

Balke B, Anthony J, Wyatt F 1989 The effects of massage treatment on exercise fatigue. Clinical Sports Medicine 1: 189–196

Barr J S, Taslitz N 1970 The influence of back massage on autonomic functions. Physical Therapy 50: 1679–1691

Beck M 1988 The theory and practice of therapeutic massage. Milady, New York

De Weaver M K 1977 Nursing home patients' perceptions of nurses' affective touching. Journal of Psychology 96: 163–171

Ferrel-Torry A T, Glick O J 1993 The use of therapeutic massage as a nursing intervention to modify anxiety and the perception of cancer pain. Cancer Nursing 16: 93–101

Field T M et al 1993 Tactile/kinaesthetic stimulation. Paediatrics 77: 654–658

Fraser J, Ross Kerr J 1993 Psychophysiological effects of back massage in elderly institutionalised patients. Journal of Advanced Nursing 18: 238–245

Hovind H, Neilsen S L 1974 Effect of massage on blood flow in skeletal muscle. Scandinavian Journal of Rehabilitation Medicine 6: 74–77

Kaada B, Torsteinbo O 1989 Increase of plasma beta endorphin levels in connective tissue massage. General Pharmacology 20: 487–489

Longworth J C D 1982 Psychophysiological effects of slow stroke massage in normotensive females. Advances in Nursing Science July: 44–46

McKecknie A A et al 1983 Anxiety states: a preliminary report on the value of connective tissue massage. Journal of Psychosomatic Research 27: 125–129

McNamarra P 1993 Massage for people with cancer. Wandsworth Cancer Support Centre, London

Morgan R G et al 1992 Complex physical therapy for the lymphoedematous arm. Journal of Hand Surgery 178: 437–441

Mortimer P S 1990 The measurement of skin lymph flow by isotope clearance — reliability, reproducibility, injection dynamics and the effect of massage. Journal of Investigative Dermatology 95: 677–681

Reed B V, Held J M 1988 Effects of sequential connective tissue massage on the autonomic nervous system of middle aged and elderly adults. Physical Therapy 68: 1231–1234

FURTHER READING – JOURNALS

Barnet K 1972 A theoretical construct of the concepts of touch as they relate to nursing. Nursing Research 21: 102–110

Jackson S 1985 The touching process in rehabilitation. Australian Nurses' Journal 14: 43–45

FURTHER READING – BOOKS

Dawes N, Harrold F 1990 Massage cures. Thorsons, Wellingborough

Maxwell-Hudson C 1988 The complete book of massage. Dorling Kindersley, London

Montague A 1986 Touching — the human significance of the skin, 3rd edn. Harper & Row, New York

USEFUL ADDRESSES

Churchill Centre
22 Montague Street
London W1H 1TB
Tel: 0171 402 9475

Clare Maxwell-Hudson's Massage
Training Centre
PO Box 457
London NW2 4ER
Tel: 0181 450 6494

Northern Institute of Massage
100 Waterloo Road
Blackpool
Lancashire FY4 1AW
Tel: 01253 403548

Raworth College for Sports Therapy
and Natural Medicines
Smallburgh
Beare Green
Dorking
Surrey RH5 4QA
Tel: 01306 712623

17 Reflexology

Pamela Griffiths

Reflexology — *a treatment which applies varying degrees of pressure to different parts of the body, usually the hands or feet, in order to promote health and well-being.*

The term 'reflexology' to some extent describes the basis of this therapy. It is suggested that there are reflexes or zones running along the body which terminate in the hands or feet. All systems and organs of the body are said to be reflected on to the surface of the skin, in particular on to the hands and feet. Thus, by applying gentle pressure to these areas it is possible to effect a change in another part of the body in order to promote well-being and relaxation. This form of therapy can influence not only specific organs but also the relationship between organs, other systems and processes (Goodwin 1988).

Depending upon the type of training undertaken by a practitioner one of several techniques may be adopted during therapy. However, the underlying principles of the different methods are consistent. These methods are as follows:

- Traditional reflexology — Bailey, Ingham (Hall 1986)
- Reflex zone therapy (Marquardt 1983)
- Metamorphic technique (Saint-Pierre & Shapiro 1989)
- Morrell method (Hewetson 1989)
- Holistic multidimensional reflexology (Ashkenazi 1993)
- Vacuflex reflexology (Dougans and Ellis 1982)

Research in reflexology

There is a vast amount of empirical but very little scientific research to support reflexology theory at present. However, some recent examples are outlined here. Flocco (1992) studied the use of reflexology in premenstrual syndrome. A total of 52 women in three groups (control, placebo reflexology and active reflexology) participated over a

6-month period. Daily diaries were maintained and once a week for 8 weeks they received treatment. The women recorded 39 separate symptoms, intensity and changes daily for six menstrual cycles. The results showed over 39% improvement in symptoms in the active group as compared with 13.8% in the placebo group.

In another study, a team of Morrell reflexologists treated 52 patients before and after knee and hip surgery. The amount of analgesia requested and given was noted, which showed that pain relief postoperatively was reduced for up to 3 days following reflexology treatment. Also, 5% of the patients treated were discharged home approximately 3 days earlier than the rest (Griffiths 1993).

HISTORICAL BACKGROUND

There is evidence to suggest that the therapeutic use of hand and foot pressure for the treatments of pain and various illnesses was in existence in China and India over 5000 years ago and was used by American Indian tribes (Goodwin 1988). A wall painting in the Egyptian tomb of Ankhmahor Saqqara 2300 BC depicts this therapy.

More recent descriptions of reflexology are commonly attributed to studies at the end of the nineteenth century by Dr William Fitzgerald, an American ear, nose and throat specialist. Fitzgerald found, quite by accident, that gentle pressure applied to specific parts of the hand or foot could cause partial local anaesthesia in areas of the ear, nose and throat. By using pressure points on the hands and feet Fitzgerald claimed to be able to perform minor surgery without conventional anaesthetics (Goodwin 1988).

Fitzgerald attempted to map the areas or zones of the hands and feet and, in 1917, in association with Dr Edwin Bowers published a treatise describing reflex zone therapy (Berkson 1977). This identified ten zones running through the body and gave maps of the internal organs reflected on the hands and feet. Fitzgerald suggested that controlled pressure with the fingers and thumbs at the end of these zones could produce a response elsewhere in the body, and that reflexology stimulated not only the organ but also the interrelationship between organs and other body systems.

In 1920, Dr Joseph Riley further developed this method and his book *Zone Therapy Simplified* describes horizontal zones of the feet (Marquardt 1983, Goodwin 1988). More recently, Eunice Ingham, a research assistant with Riley, further refined the theory and attempted to define precise zone pathways. Ingham maintains that by focusing on foot pressure, all parts of the body may be treated (Booth 1993). In the early 1960s, Doreen Bailey met Ingham whilst in America and upon her return to the UK, began to practise and encourage interest in reflexology here.

The concept of channels of energy flowing around the body is not unique to reflexology; therapeutic touch, acupuncture and shiatsu are based on similar theories of an innate body energy that can be treated on the body surface to stimulate internal organs. Dougans & Ellis (1992) suggest that reflexology, like acupuncture, works with the meridians but much more research on these 'energy pathways' is needed.

TREATMENT

Reflexology suggests that every part of the body is connected by reflex zones or pathways terminating in the soles of the feet, palms of the hands, ears, tongue and head (Corvo 1990, Ashkenazi 1993). The reflex zones relate to all areas of the body through ten longitudinal zones, which are symmetrical with five on each side of the body.

It is suggested that tension, congestion or some other imbalance will affect the whole zone and that it is possible to treat one part of the zone, such as the foot, to bring about a change in other specified parts of the body (Barron 1990). Ingham considered that malfunction of any organ or part of the body resulted in tiny crystalline deposits of calcium and uric acid on the nerve endings of the feet (Goodwin 1988). Gentle pressure is thought to facilitate the breakdown and elimination of these deposits and so promote health and well-being (Ingham 1938). This is referred to as detoxification and the signs that it is occurring as a 'healing crisis'. Once this process has occurred, healing can begin.

The foot is treated by applying gentle pressure along each zone systematically until the entire foot has been covered. This includes the dorsum, sides and top – then the same process is carried out on the other foot. Initially, gentle massage and stroking movements are used, followed by deep thumb and finger pressures. If there is an imbalance or blockage of energy in any of the zones or reflexes, they may feel tender or painful and gentle pressures are applied to remove the blockage. Reflex treatment is said to treat the body on a number of levels simultaneously: the sole of the foot has areas relating to specific organs and also to the emotions. The treatment can influence emotional, physical and spiritual disorders (Goodwin 1988).

After treatment, a healing crisis may occur due to detoxification of the body (Sahai 1993). Some examples of healing crisis symptoms are as follows:

- 'Flu-like' symptoms
- Feeling light-headed, very relaxed
- Feeling very cold 3–4 days post-treatment
- Increase in excretory functions
- Reduction in blood pressure
- Lethargy
- Enhanced or altered sleep pattern.

It is essential that nurses are aware of and able to manage symptoms of a reflexology healing crisis, as distinct from pathological conditions, and know when to refer to other health care practitioners. Thus, a good training course is recommended before using reflexology in professional practice.

Training in reflexology

This technique may be harmful if not used correctly, despite the popular belief that it is a simple foot massage. There is no current governing body for training and there are several schools with varying course length, student numbers and standards. The courses should be a minimum of one year, and preferably affiliated to a professional body such as the British Register of Health Practitioners or the Association of Reflexologists (AR). The AR, founded in 1984, aims to monitor and maintain standards of professional practice. Nurses can also consult the Royal College of Nursing Special Interest Group Guidelines on Complementary Therapy Courses (RCNSIG 1993).

Types of treatment

Some of the techniques based on traditional zone therapy, are outlined next.

Holistic reflexology

Morrell and holistic multidimensional reflexology treatments last about 30 minutes and use the same zone theory but mirror image each move from foot to foot, rather than zone to zone, using ultra-gentle palpation of the feet. Alterations in skin tone and texture are identified and all imbalances of the feet are painlessly treated with minimum healing crisis reaction. This is due to the resultant deep relaxation; respiratory rate, pulse and heart rate are decreased, blood pressure is homoeostatically balanced, and stimulation of healing energies is achieved (Dougans & Ellis 1992). Owing to these physiological changes, homoeostasis can be regained and maintained. This results in relief of symptoms, and facilitates the rebuilding and rebalancing of energies required to aid healing and prevent illness. The author whilst taking part in a pilot study on orthopaedic patients, found that after treatment most patients were more relaxed, in less pain and able to sleep better.

Metamorphic technique

This approach was developed by Robert St John in the 1960s, working on the theory that the foot mirrors the 9-month gestation period in utero and that problems that develop in utero go on to later life. Early therapy may remove the problems. The feet, hands and head are gently rubbed to relieve the pressure said to be causing blockages in energy flow (Gonzales & Saint-Pierre 1992).

Vacuflex reflexology

This is a two-phase treatment linking reflex stimulation and meridian rebalancing. Specially developed suction boots are put on the feet and suction cups in specific areas of the body stimulate the reflexes, when connected to a suction pump. The theory combines reflexology, acupressure and cupping to bring about homoeostasis (Dougans & Ellis 1982).

Therapeutic potential in nursing

Reflexology offers a wide range of potential benefits for nurses practising within a multidisciplinary team in all health sectors. Maternity and care of the elderly are showing particular interest in this therapy. Many conditions and ages may be treated by qualified therapists. Most conditions respond within a few sessions, depending on the individual. Note, however, that not everyone will find the intensity of the treatment acceptable. Therapeutic benefits include:

■ Pain relief in acute and chronic states

■ Control of anxiety

■ Reduction in blood pressure, pulse, temperature and hormone levels, thereby improving circulation, breathing and elimination

■ Deep relaxation

- Detoxification
- Revitalizing and rebalancing effects, facilitating healing
- Immune system strengthening
- Improved (rapid eye movement) sleep
- Preventive measure as part of health promotion
- Wound healing.

Treatment should only be carried out by a trained practitioner and preferably as part of a multidisciplinary approach. Cross-professional referring of clients ensures the most effective system of care.

Contraindications for use

- Some individuals may find the intensity of this therapy unacceptable.
- It is not generally used for diagnosis, except in preventive health care (Morrell or holistic multidimensional reflexology).
- For some conditions, e.g. diabetes and hyper/hypothyroidism, the reflexologist must work closely with medical colleagues.
- Reflexology it is not suitable for the first trimester of pregnancy.
- It should be used cautiously with patients in depressive and manic states.
- Use with care in epilepsy and in acute conditions.

Summary

Reflexology is potentially a very valuable therapeutic nursing skill and could have wide-ranging and cost-effective benefits in health care, from special care baby units through to care of the elderly. Like many other complementary therapies, reflexology seems to restore and maintain health by rebalancing the body. Whilst to many, reflexology may appear a gentle therapy, it is vital that the contraindications are known and that it is only carried out by trained therapists.

REFERENCES

Ashkenazi R 1993 Multidimensional reflexology. International Journal of Alternative and Complementary Medicine June: 8–12
Barron H 1990 Towards better health with reflexology. Nursing Standard 4: 32–33

Berkson D 1977 The foot book — healing the body through reflexology. Barnes & Nobles, New York

Booth B 1993 Complementary therapy. Nursing Times/Macmillan, London

Booth B 1994 Reflexology. Nursing Times 5: 38–40

Corvo J 1990 Zone therapy. Century, London

Dougans I, Ellis S 1992 The art of reflexology. Element, Dorset

Flocco B 1992 Reflexology and pre menstrual syndrome research study. Reflections 6–9

Gonzales M A, Saint-Pierre G 1992 Any difference between reflexology and the metamorphic technique? Metamorphosis 26: 69–71

Goodwin H 1988 Reflex zone therapy cited in Rankin-Box D (ed) Complementary health therapies: a guide for nurses and the caring professions. Chapman and Hall, London

Griffiths P 1993 Tickling innovation in Cardiff. Full House Conference Report Orthopaedic Bare Bone No 20 Autumn newsletter. Society of Orthopaedic Nursing, Royal College of Nursing. Smith and Nephew, London

Hall N M 1986 Reflexology: a patients guide. Thorsons, Wellingborough

Hewetson R 1989 Feet first. Haps (Chepstow), Bristol

Ingham E 1938 Stories the feet can tell. Ingham, St Petersburg, Florida

Marquardt H 1983 Reflex zone therapy of the feet. Thorsons, Wellingborough

Sahai I C M 1993 Reflexology — its place in modern health care. Professional Nurse 18: 722–725

FURTHER READING

Bayley D E 1982 Reflexology today (revised edn). Thorsons, Wellingborough

Kunz K, Kunz B 1986 Hand and foot reflexology. Thorsons, Wellingborough

Norman L, Cowan T 1989 The reflexology handbook. Piatkus, London

Richards W J 1990 Sole searching. Here's Health 34: 37

USEFUL ADDRESSES

Association of Reflexologists
27 Old Gloucester Street
London WC1 3XX
Tel: 0171 237 6523

Association of Vacuflex
Reflexologists
25 Meadowcroft Close
East Grinstead
West Sussex RNH19 1NA
Tel: 01342 24019

British Reflexology Association
Monks Orchard
Whitbourne
Worcester WR6 5RB
Tel: 01886 212707

British School — Reflex Zone
Therapy of the Feet
87 Oakington Avenue
Wembley Park
London HA9 8HY
Tel: 0181 908 2201

Holistic Association of British
Reflexologists
92 Sheering Road
Old Harrow
Essex CM17 0JW
Tel: 01279 429060

Institute of Complementary
Medicine
PO Box 194
London SE14 1QZ

Metamorphic Association
67 Ritherdon Road
London SW17 8QE
Tel: 0181 6725951

Rose Cottage Complementary
Living Centre
Clun Avenue
Pontyclun
Midglamorgan CF7 9AG
Tel: 01443 229190

18 Relaxation and visualization

Lynne Ryman

Relaxation — *a state of consciousness characterized by feelings of peace and release from tension, anxiety and fear.*

Visualization — *using the imagination to create desired changes in an individual's life.*

Relaxation and visualization are planned and structured activities leading to peace of mind and enhanced quality of life (Ryman 1994). In this respect, successful practice of relaxation and visualization techniques can result in the ability to control and reduce tension, worry and anxiety (Ryman 1994). It is well-accepted and documented that excessive stress interferes with a person's well-being and ability to enjoy life (Friedman et al 1969, Selye 1976). Where tension is experienced over long periods of time this may have a depressing effect on the immune system leading to ill-health and disease (Ryman 1994). For total health and happiness all aspects of human experience, emotional, physical, mental, psychological and spiritual, need to be in a balanced state and in harmony with each other; disease can occur when they are not (Simonton et al 1978).

Relaxation and visualization work together to provide a therapy which encourages negative unhealthy states of mind to be replaced by positive healthy ones. The role of relaxation is to bring the mind of the participant to a state of balance and peace. Visualization uses this balanced state to remove negative or self-destructive thoughts and move towards a better state, as perceived by the client. Relaxation and visualization can facilitate health-giving changes, such as getting well again, losing weight, stopping smoking, staying well, etc.

Relaxation and visualization provide a necessary and healing break in the daily routine; they are strategies for self-healing and illness prevention when used regularly. Relaxation of body, mind and spirit is one way in which to regain and maintain a healthy, harmonious, whole human being (Ryman 1994).

HISTORICAL BACKGROUND

The many ways in which people can learn to reduce levels of stress are well documented. Throughout history peace of mind has been gained by repetitive praying (teaching the mind to dwell on one thought) and by meditation (Benson & Klipper 1977). One of the first modern techniques developed for stress reduction was 'progressive relaxation' (Jacobson 1977), based on the idea that muscle tension or relaxation influences the state of the entire person. In progressive relaxation, the person tenses and then relaxes successive groups of muscles, focusing attention on the differences experienced when muscles are in a tense or relaxed state (Ryman 1994). Jacobson's technique entailed learning to relax 218 different muscle groups and required perseverance and time to master successfully.

The relaxation response devised by Benson in 1974 is a simpler process that almost anyone can use. It requires the following:

- A quiet environment
- A word or phrase repeated over and over again
- The adoption of a passive attitude
- A comfortable position.

Regular practice should promote a markedly enhanced state of well-being (Benson & Klipper 1977, Ryman 1994). At first Benson felt that the four basic components listed were essential. Subsequently he specified just two:

- Repetition of a word, a sound, a prayer, a phrase or a muscular movement
- Passive disregard of everyday thoughts when they occur.

Other techniques used to achieve a relaxed state include autogenic training, biofeedback, hypnosis and slow stroke massage, to mention but a few.

Visualization is the use of mental imaging to alleviate and prevent disease. This practice has been documented throughout history and is commonly associated with American and African shamanism. Some oriental therapies also made use of visualization (Reader's Digest 1991, Ryman 1994). Since the early 1970s the names of Carl and Stephanie Simonton (Simonton 1978) have become synonymous with visualization following their extensive use of this method in working with severe illness, such as cancer. The subject is taught to focus on an appropriate image, preferably of their choice, to induce a feeling of peace or happiness or to promote beneficial changes in health or circumstance.

Relaxation and visualization methods are being increasingly researched world-wide, to discover whether and how states of mind can influence physiological changes in the body and psychological well-being (Meares 1979, Patel et al 1985, Chang 1991).

TREATMENT

Everyone has an innate self-protective mechanism against too much stress. This 'relaxation response' (Benson & Klipper 1977) is characterized by decreased heart rate, lowered metabolism, decreased rate of breathing and slower brain waves, which help return the body to a healthier balanced state.

As part of a structured programme to promote health-giving, deep breathing and progressive muscle relaxation techniques can be used on their own or for greater benefit in combination with visualization. The basic technique (Ryman 1994) is outlined next.

Participants sit comfortably with eyes closed, feet firmly fixed on the floor, spine supported and fingers and feet uncrossed. The session usually lasts for 30 to 45 minutes and the theme of self-awareness and seeing oneself in one's mind's eye is encouraged throughout. There are generally three parts to the session in the following order:

- Observation of the normal breathing pattern, its rate, rhythm and depth, followed by deeper breathing.

- Progressive muscle relaxation — tensing and relaxing major muscle groups throughout the body paying particular attention to sensing the opposite poles of tension and relaxation.

- The visualization exercise, in which participants are first encouraged to experience, for example, a country walk with all their senses (sight, touch, smell, taste, hearing). From the peaceful state achieved by this, they move on to more specific visualizations designed to address current issues, for example:

   — a war waged between good cells and diseased cells (with the good cells winning)

   — picturing a laser beam destroying tissue affected by disease (and leaving good tissue free)

   — seeing in every detail a desired scenario, such as being full of well-being, wholeness and happiness

—an improved relationship
—being free of pain.

Researchers now believe that the images used in the visualization above should be chosen by the individuals themselves, since they are more likely to be relevant and therefore effective (Simonton 1978). Good images are subjective and unique, in line with the individualistic approach of many complementary therapies.

It is very important that on completion of the exercise each participant is well grounded before resuming normal activity. Regular practice is necessary, since a cumulative effect gives the best results. Tapes for home use are helpful.

Stages of technique

Stage I
—normal level of consciousness
—full awareness
—beta brain wave, characterized by decision-making, reasoning and logic
—emotions: full range

Stage II
—changed level of consciousness
—relaxed mellowness
—alpha brain wave, characterized by a lessening effect of negative thoughts and feelings
—emotions: stilled, muted

Stage III
—changed level of consciousness
—very lucid: intense alertness
—alpha/theta or alpha/beta, characterized by openness to ideas of creativity, inspiration and healing
—emotions; calmness and detachment; deeply satisfying

Therapeutic potential in nursing

A growing number of hospitals now offer on a regular basis relaxation and visualization to their staff and patients in the form of self-help groups. Below are some of the benefits:

- Hypertension: a non-pharmacological way of reducing high blood pressure (mild, acute and chronic)

- Insomnia: aids return to a normal sleep pattern, leading to reaffirmation of homoeostasis

- Coronary artery disease: provides a way for reversing heart disease without the use of drugs or surgery
- Arthritis: lessens pain/disabilities; aids regression of disease
- Stress management: reduces levels of tension, anxiety and stress, leading to a more balanced outlook on life
- Potentially painful procedures: through self-awareness and self-control decreases distress and discomfort without sedation
- Immune system: strengthens to give less susceptibility to disease
- Pain, management of all forms: reduction with relaxation alone but increased efficiency when used with visualization
- Positive outlook: lessens negativity and renews hope; allows clients to take part in their own healing
- Reduction in side effects such as nausea and vomiting caused by radiotherapy, chemotherapy; decreased analgesia post-operatively
- Cancer: can help to reduce anger, anxiety and depression caused by trauma of disease
- Relaxation: facilitates peace of mind and insight into the nature of one's problems and the influence of attitude in dealing with these issues
- Coping mechanisms: increases ability to cope, re-energizes, leads to an improvement in quality of life
- Panic attacks: can reduce fear and lead to reduction of symptoms and an understanding of the cause of anxiety.

Contraindications for use

- Subjects may have difficulty acquiring the skill.
- It may be fatiguing for the weak or ill since sustained concentration is required to elicit the response.
- Patients with dyspnoea may not respond to a focus on breathing.
- Patients with cardiac irregularities may experience increased irregularity.
- Patients with low back pain may benefit more from strengthening their muscles rather than relaxing them.
- If used for more than two periods of 20–30 minutes daily some may experience withdrawal from life and symptoms ranging from insomnia to hallucinations.
- Psychotic patients may decompensate with profound relaxation
- Allergic or other adverse reactions may result if certain triggers are activated, e.g. picturing a corn field for a patient with hay fever.

Summary

The relaxation response is generally believed to have few if any negative effects, especially when relaxation is combined with visualization and providing both are competently taught and carried out. Perhaps the most cost-effective of all the complementary therapies, relaxation and visualization encourage patients to develop a sense of well-being and self-awareness. Self-healing results and the therapy can lead to personal development and growth.

REFERENCES

Benson H, Klipper M Z 1977 The relaxation response. Collins, London

Chang J 1991 Using relaxation strategies in child and youth care practice. Child and Youth Care Forum 20: 155–169

Friedman S B, Glasgow L A, Ader R 1969 Psychosocial factors modifying host resistance to experimental infections. Annals of the New York Academy of Sciences 164: 381–393

Jacobson E 1977 You must relax, 5th edn. Souvenir Press, London

Meares A 1979 Strange places, simple truths. Collins, Glasgow

Patel C, Marmot M G, Terry D J et al 1985 Trial of relaxation in reducing coronary risk: four year follow up. British Medical Journal 290 (6475): 1103–1106

Reader's Digest Association 1991 Visualisation therapy; picturing your way to health. In: Reader's Digest family guide to alternative medicine. Reader's Digest Association, London

Ryman L 1994 Relaxation and visualisation. In: Wells R J, Tschudin V (eds) Wells' supportive therapies in health care. Baillière Tindall, London

Selye H 1976 The stress of life, revised edn. McGraw-Hill, New York

Simonton O C, Matthews-Simonton S, Creighton J L 1978 Getting well again, a step-by-step, self-help guide to overcoming cancer for patients and their families. Bantam, London

FURTHER READING – JOURNALS

Asaenok I S, Spetsian L M, Laysha N A 1988 Experience in using rooms for psycho-emotional relaxation at an engineering plant. Gigiena Truda i Professionalnye Zabolevaniia Jun 6: 50–51

Relaxation was found markedly to reduce the high fatigue levels felt at the end of the shift and also to bring about considerable reduction of the levels of irritation felt at work and disturbed sleep patterns.

Bullock E A, Shaddy R E 1993 Relaxation and imagery techniques without sedation during right ventricular endomyocardial biopsy in pediatric heart transplant patients. Journal of Heart and Lung Transplantation 12: 59–62

Butler R J 1993 Establishing a dry run; a case study in securing bladder control. British Journal of Clinical Psychology 39: 215–217

Decker T W, Cline-Elsen J 1992 Relaxation therapy as an adjunct in radiation oncology. Journal of Clinical Psychology 48: 388–393

Engel J M, Rapoff M A, Pressman A R 1992 Long-term follow-up of relaxation training for pediatric headache disorders. Headache 32: 152–156

Konno Y, Ohno K 1987 A factor analytic study of the acceptance of relaxation through Dohsa training (psychological rehabilitation training). Shinrigaku Kenkyu (Japanese Journal of Psychology) 58: 57–61
This indicated amongst other things that willingness to apply oneself to the relaxation technique is indispensable for the required change.

Litchfield J 1993 Visualisation in coronary artery disease. Care of the Critically Ill 9: 35–36

Patel C, Marmot M G, Terry D J et al 1985 Trial of relaxation in reducing coronary risk: four year follow up. British Medical Journal 290 (6475): 1103–1106

Stephens R L 1992 Imagery: a treatment for nursing student anxiety. Journal of Nursing Education 31: 314–320

Zachariae R, Kristensen J S, Hokland P et al 1990 Effect of psychological intervention in the form of relaxation and guided imagery on cellular immune function in normal healthy subjects. An overview. Psychotherapy and Psychosomatics 54: 32–39

FURTHER READING – BOOKS

Chaitow L 1985 Your complete stress-proofing programme; how to protect yourself against the ill-effects of stress, including relaxation and meditation techniques. Thorsons, Wellingborough

Fleming U 1990 Grasping the nettle: a positive approach to pain. Collins Fount Paperbacks, London
Looks at the problem of pain in various forms (physical, mental and emotional) and shows a new way of learning how to live with it and overcome it.

Gawain S 1982 Creative visualisation. Bantam, New York
An introduction and work-book for the art of using mental energy to transform and greatly improve health, prosperity and loving relationships.

Madders J 1987 Stress and relaxation; self-help ways to cope with stress and relieve nervous tension, ulcers, insomnia, migraine and high blood pressure, 3rd edn. Macdonald Optima, London

Markham U 1989 The elements of visualisation. Element, Dorset
Describes visualization and looks at what it can do, what techniques are involved and how it can help improve our lives.

USEFUL ADDRESSES

There is no governing body or national register of relaxation and visualization therapists. The Relaxation for Living Foundation (see below) provides courses for those wishing to learn to relax (using mainly physical exercise methods) and for those who wish to go on to teach others. A recent and exciting venture for nurses is an ENB course (see below) on stress management which has as one of its components relaxation.

British Holistic Medical Association (BHMA)
179 Gloucester Place
London NW1 6DX
Tel: 0171 262 5299

English National Board for Nursing, Midwifery and Health Visiting (ENB)
170 Tottenham Court Road
London W1P 9LG
Stress management course for nurses.

International Stress and Tension Control Society (UK Branch)
The Priory Hospital
Priory Lane
Roehampton
London SW15 5JQ
Tel: 0181 876 8261

Relaxation for Living
168–170 Oatlands Drive
Weybridge
Surrey KT13 9ET
Runs classes in London and most parts of the country.

19 Shiatsu

Caroline Stevensen

Shiatsu — a hands-on therapy which works on energetic pathways to balance and strengthen the body.

'Shiatsu' means 'finger pressure' in Japanese but in practice is much more than that. It is a therapy performed by the use of pressure from fingers, hands, elbows, knees and feet on the energetic pathways of the body called 'meridians'. It is along these meridians that the vital energy or life force of the body, known as 'Ki', flows. Shiatsu aims to harmonize the Ki, promoting health and well-being throughout body, mind and spirit. It is traditionally performed on a padded mat or futon with the recipient clothed.

Shiatsu has its roots in oriental medicine and massage techniques dating back over 2000 years. The modern form of shiatsu was introduced to the west only in the last 25 years (Gulliver et al 1993). It is a therapy which can be preventive as well as helpful in specific conditions. Through balancing the Ki, the recipient experiences relaxation and an improvement in many health problems. Shiatsu is a complementary therapy that can be given in conjunction with orthodox medical treatments as well as being a therapy in its own right. It combines diagnostic and treatment methods and encourages self-healing. It is being used increasingly in a wide variety of settings, but to date few nurses have undergone training.

HISTORICAL BACKGROUND

Massage, herbalism, acupuncture and moxibustion are all part of traditional Chinese medicine. The initial practice of massage in Japan known as 'Anma' resembles current western massage in its active movements. Shiatsu, however, developed as a more subtle art involving the giving of still, relaxed pressure at defined points over the body (Lundberg 1992). It emerged from a manual therapy incorporating gentle manipulation, stretches and pressure techniques. It was recognized by the Japanese government as a therapy in its own right in the middle of the twentieth century (Lundberg 1992) and was brought to Europe, USA, Australia and other parts of the western world over the last 25 years where it is increasingly being used alongside orthodox health care.

Shiatsu is based on the 2000-year-old philosophy of traditional Chinese medicine (TCM). This states that from the universe or 'Tao', life energy made itself manifest in the forces of Yin and Yang, the positive and negative aspects of Ki. Ki flows through the body, supporting life and all its functions. The theory of Yin and Yang, the balance of opposite but complementary forces, was extended to include the Five Elements or Phases — Wood, Fire, Earth, Metal and Water — which influence the flow of Ki. On the basis of this complex system, definite characteristics were identified and associated with conditions of the body, illnesses or imbalances (Beresford Cooke 1987). For example, the shouting quality in the voice and florid complexion of an alcoholic are related to disharmony in the Liver, ruled by the Wood element. TCM recognizes spiritual, mental, emotional and physical causes of disease and takes into account factors such as diet, exercise and other external influences, including climate. (See Chapter 6 on Acupuncture for further information on TCM theory.) Ki flows along the meridians defined in TCM and there have been some studies to support the existence of these energetic pathways (Becker 1976).

Styles of shiatsu

Various styles of shiatsu are practised in Japan and the West. These include zen shiatsu (most common), macrobiotic shiatsu, healing shiatsu, Namikoshi shiatsu and hara shiatsu (Gulliver et al 1993). The general principles previously mentioned apply to all approaches.

TREATMENT

Zen shiatsu, involves the following sequence of events:

- History of the patient and his condition
- Diagnosis performed on the hara (abdomen) or back
- Delivery of the treatment

- Reassessment of the hara or back
- Recommendations to the patient.

History of the patient and his condition

A medical history of the patient is taken which includes any illnesses and operations, medications, acute and chronic conditions and the patient's response to external factors such as food, weather, seasons of the year, times of the day and night, energy levels, general mood and, in the case of women, menstrual problems. The person's colouring, voice, posture and general attitude are also noted. Tongue and pulse diagnosis may be performed for a fuller understanding of the patient according to TCM.

Positioning of the patient

Shiatsu treatment is traditionally performed on a futon on the floor but can be given in a sitting position or on a treatment couch if the patient has difficulty getting down to floor level. A lower position makes it easier for the practitioner to provide pressure perpendicular to the meridian pathways with the help of gravity. The patient is fully clothed, preferably in a cotton tracksuit and socks. With the patient lying on his back, supported where necessary by pillows, the practitioner can observe the body for areas of tension and weakness. Any imbalance of Ki in the meridians as well as potential and existing health problems may be observed.

Diagnosis performed on the hara or back

Shiatsu diagnosis is performed on the hara (abdomen) or back by gentle palpation. The relative energetic qualities of the internal organs and their related meridians are assessed. Between the weakest, empty or most 'kyo' and the tightest, fullest or most 'jitsu' meridian, a reaction is felt by the practitioner which then guides the treatment.

Delivery of the treatment

The principles in giving zen shiatsu are as follows (Masunaga & Ohashi 1997):

- Stationary perpendicular pressure: direct pressure is exerted at 90° to the meridian pathway.

- Penetration not pressure: pressure is exerted on the meridian point leaning with body weight and the help of gravity (not by physical force).
- Two-handed connectedness: both hands are used, one for support and the other to treat the meridian.
- Meridian continuity: the meridian is treated in its entirety to relieve any Ki blocked along its pathway and to give support as necessary.
- Relaxation of practitioner achieved by linking mind, hara and breath.

Intention and motivation are as important in shiatsu as any other therapy. The focus of shiatsu is at the point on the hara called 'Tandem', the centre of balance and gravity, which is one centimetre below the umbilicus (Jarmey & Tschudin 1994). Shiatsu given from this point is relaxing and centring for the practitioner as well as the patient.

In shiatsu, treatment concentrates on the most kyo meridian, rather like supporting the weakest link in a chain. To begin, the 'supporting' hand is placed on the hara whilst the other hand 'palms' the leg along the weakest meridian pathway, feeling for imbalances in the Ki. The process is then repeated with the thumb, fingers, elbow or knee leaning in along the same meridian in order to balance the Ki. Along the meridians there are highly charged electromagnetic foci called 'tsubos' or pressure points (Ridolfi 1990) (these correspond to acupuncture points). The stimulation of the tsubos affects the meridian energy as well as energy in other parts of the body. By feeling the changing quality of the Ki along the meridian and in the tsubos the appropriate amount of pressure can be given to balance the energy. This process can then be repeated systematically around the body until the entire meridian system has been treated. The pressure of shiatsu should be deep but not overly painful. Blocked energy in a tsubo may feel painful and sensitive. Low energy may be felt deeper in the body. Recipients often describe a 'good hurt' in places where treatment is particularly needed. Pressures and stretches to other meridians are included in the treatment as appropriate. The whole body is worked on including the front, back, sides, limbs, neck and head, again according to individual need.

Reassessment of the hara or back

Following treatment, the hara or back is reassessed by gentle palpation to detect changes and improvement in the 'distribution of Ki' or energetic balance. People commonly feel both invigorated and relaxed after shiatsu. An overall improvement in health and well-being is often felt before any change in a chronic condition. The eliminative channels of the body may need to be cleared before pain can be alleviated. Improvements on the physical, mental, emotional and spiritual levels are achieved with shiatsu. As with other such therapies, a 'healing reaction' may be provoked (Gulliver 1993). Long-standing stress, tension or a build-up of toxins may be released in the form of a slight aggravation of the condition or possibly 'flu like symptoms. This usually passes in less than 48 hours and an improvement is then felt.

Recommendations to the patient

Recommendations may include diet, exercise and lifestyle changes based on traditional Chinese medicine theory for the overall improvement of health, according to the individual.

Therapeutic potential in nursing

The main aims of shiatsu are as follows (Jarmey & Tschudin 1994):
- To promote relaxation
- To improve blood and lymphatic flow
- To alleviate aches and pains
- To provide empathy and support
- To heighten bodily awareness.

The conditions most amenable to treatment by shiatsu and of therapeutic benefit in nursing are (Ridolfi 1990):
- headaches and migraine
- respiratory illnesses including asthma and bronchitis
- sinus trouble with catarrh
- insomnia and restlessness
- circulatory problems
- anxiety and tension
- depression and other psychological problems
- fatigue and lethargy
- somatic disturbances resulting from mental problems
- digestive disorders

- bowel problems
- low libido
- painful menstruation
- pregnancy and childbirth
- urogenital conditions
- rheumatic and arthritic complaints
- back trouble, including sciatica
- following sprains and strains and other injuries, but not in first 24 hours due to pain and swelling
- integration of physical, mental, emotional and spiritual aspects.

To say that shiatsu can be helpful for any condition may be a little broad but certainly in improving overall well-being, promoting calm, rest and relaxation, it can enhance quality of life for most people. Indeed, shiatsu can be ideal for maintaining good health. Although conditions are treated according to oriental diagnosis with shiatsu, western medical diagnosis can be taken into account.

Contraindications for use

As shiatsu works directly on the body, the contraindications for general massage apply. Do not treat:

- Osteoporosis, fractures and bony metastases due to pressure
- Burns, wounds, broken skin, infectious skin diseases
- Unexplained swellings
- Operation sites for at least 1–2 months
- Directly over varicose veins
- Low platelet count, tendency to easy bruising, over present bruising
- High fevers, as touch is generally not tolerated
- Contagious diseases due to infection risk
- Lower legs and specifically contraindicated points in the first trimester of pregnancy, especially if there is a history of spontaneous abortion
- Immune deficiency problems including AIDS, ME and cancer; lighter techniques and shorter treatments may be used so as not to exhaust the patient
- Cardiac or chronic respiratory patients in the prone position, unless an exact knowledge of their current status is known
- On the head with epileptics or with blood pressure > 200 mmHg systolic

Summary

Shiatsu is a deep and effective hands-on treatment for many conditions as well as being very relaxing and providing support for general health and well-being. Through the balancing of the body's energy, better physiological and psychological functioning can occur. Recommendations for diet and lifestyle based on TCM theory can also be offered, according to individual need. The 3-year part-time training in shiatsu is demanding but enables the nurse using shiatsu to offer a particularly beneficial complementary therapy.

REFERENCES

Becker R, Marino A, Spadaro J 1976 Electrophysiological correlates of acupuncture points and meridians. Psychoenergetic Systems 1: 105–112
Beresford Cooke C 1987 Shiatsu. In: Lidell L (ed) The book of massage. Ebury Press, London
Gulliver N, Liechti E, Lunberg P 1993 A guide to shiatsu. Shiatsu Society, Wokingham
Jarmey C, Tschudin V 1994 Shiatsu. In: Wells R, Tschudin V (eds) Wells' supportive therapies in health care. Baillière Tindall, London
Lundberg P 1992 The book of shiatsu. Gaia Books, London
Masunaga S, Ohashi W 1977 Zen shiatsu. Japan Publications, New York
Ridolfi R 1990 Alternative health: shiatsu. Optima, London

FURTHER READING – BOOKS

Jarmey C, Tindall J 1991 Acupressure for common ailments. Gaia Books, London
Kaptchuk T J 1989 Chinese medicine: the web that has no weaver. Rider, London
Maciocia G 1989 The foundations of Chinese medicine. Churchill Livingstone, London
Ohashi W 1988 Do-it-yourself shiatsu. Unwin Paperbacks, London

USEFUL ADDRESSES

British School of Shiatsu-Do
6 Erskine Road
London NW3 3AJ
Tel: 0171 483 3776

European Shiatsu School
Highbanks, Lockeridge
Marlborough
Wilts SN8 4EQ
Tel: 01672 86 362

Shiatsu College
20A Lower Goat Lane
Norwich NR1 2EL
(classes in London)
Tel: 01603 632555

Shiatsu Society
5 Foxcote
Wokingham
Berkshire RG11 3PG
Tel: 01734 730 836

Zen School of Shiatsu
Healing Tao Centre
2nd floor, East–West Centre
188 Old Street
London EC1
Tel: 0181 766 7636

20 Therapeutic touch

Jean Sayre-Adams

Therapeutic touch — *an energy field interaction between two or more people, aimed at rebalancing or repatterning the energy field to promote relaxation and pain relief and activate self-healing.*

The use of touch in the act of laying on of hands is one of the oldest therapies known to humans. Therapeutic touch (TT) is a modern form of the laying on of hands, and the name originates from Dr Dolores Kreiger, Professor of Nursing at New York University. The concepts that form its foundations are both simple and complex and can be found at the cutting edge of modern physics (Capra 1976, Booth 1993).

The theoretical concepts underpinning TT have been linked to the eastern ideas of chakras and meridians (Govinda 1974, Krieger 1993). More recently the theoretical basis of TT has become closely associated with Martha Rogers' theory of nursing practice — the Science of Unitary Human Beings (Rogers 1970) and consequently with relativity theory and quantum theory (Lutjens 1991). Rogers' Science of Unitary Human Beings appears to have originated approximately 30 years ago in her early writings (Lutjens 1991). She perceived nursing as a unique science, conceptually distinct from any other science. The Science of Unitary Human Beings is described as a synthesis of facts and ideas to create a unique way of perceiving people and their environment. The fulcrum of the theory is the uniqueness of human beings and their interactions with the world. This focus upon individuals is presented as underpinning the practice of nursing.

Lutjens (1991) describes Rogers' central theme as that of acausality in an infinite universe of open systems; i.e. there is no such thing as cause-and-effect since this implies a beginning and an end. In contrast to a linear approach to health care, Rogers views existence and our interactions with all things as being in a continual state of change. Drawing on Heisenberg's principle of uncertainty and on quantum theory she describes our world as an energy system. This energy is never stable but in continual flow and ebb — creating and recreating patterns, oscillating between balance and imbalance, health and illness. Human beings are seen as dynamic energy fields. Rogers' theory is continually evolving and developing but the basis of this approach is briefly as follows:

- Energy — energy fields are the fundamental units of all living things (Rogers 1990).

- Human beings are whole entities and should never be perceived simply in terms of their parts.

- Humans are energy fields and are continually and simultaneously exchanging energy with one another and with the environment.

- Each energy field has a unique pattern, rather like a finger print.

- Individual energy fields are in a continual process of interaction with the environment. Thus, even a repeated action is not the same; time has moved on and our energy has imperceptibly altered. One never walks the same stream twice (Lutjens 1990).

- Each energy field is unique though constantly changing, like a wave in the sea.

- The energy field extends to many other dimensions in addition to the three-dimensional world; this is referred to as 'pandimensionality'.

In recent years there have been suggestions that the Science of Unitary Human Beings is congruent with TT and Rogers' approach is increasingly referred to when explaining therapeutic touch. Therapeutic touch works on the premiss that all individuals are unique energy fields. Imbalances or disruptions in the flow of energy can be rebalanced or repatterned by the therapist towards a state of harmony and balance. Therapeutic touch is a specific therapeutic modality and is distinct from any other forms of energy healing (Quinn 1993).

Although there has been much research on therapeutic touch (Quinn 1988), it is still not clearly understood how therapeutic touch works. Quinn (1992) suggests a repatterning of the energy field of the person in imbalance is being initiated by the therapist, and influenced by the therapist's centred state and energy field.

HISTORICAL BACKGROUND

Although therapeutic touch is a relatively new modality, healing through touch is probably as old as civilization itself. Evidence of the use of touch to promote well-being can be found in cave drawings. The oldest written documentation of healing touch comes from the Orient 5000 years ago. It has been used in all cultures: Egyptian, Chinese, Indian, Polynesian, native American Indian, Greek and Roman (Turton 1988, Booth 1993, Harvey 1983). The Bible tells of healing through touch performed by Christ (Turton 1988). Touch was widely used by shamans and traditional practitioners until the rise of the Puritan culture during the 1600s. With the development of Christianity, Turton (1988) notes that healing was claimed as the domain of the clergy and this restricted widespread use. Touch as a healing art remained relatively unacknowledged until research into its benefits began in the 1950s (Dossey et al 1988).

In the late 1960s, Dr Dolores Krieger, Professor of Nursing at New York University, learned the laying on of hands from Dora Kunz (Kunz 1991) and over the next several years practised and promoted therapeutic touch within nursing. In the early 1970s, Krieger began to teach TT to her Masters degree students in a class entitled 'Frontiers in nursing'.

TREATMENT

The aim of a TT treatment is to rebalance or repattern the energy field of the patient, therefore bringing relaxation and facilitating the healing process. TT can be carried out in any setting that the practitioner feels is appropriate, for example, a quiet room in a hospital, in a garden, or at home. First, the practitioner centres him- or herself, in order to become harmonious with the patient. At this time the intention to help is also reaffirmed. An assessment of the patient is then made by the practitioner by moving her hands over the entire energy field. The practitioner returns to the areas where an imbalance has been felt and, continuing to use the hands, rebalances or repatterns the field.

Stages of technique

Centring — the practitioner becomes relaxed, calm and focused on the care about to be given.

Assessment — the practitioner places her hands close to the client's body and gently moves them over the body. The aim is to identify subtle changes in the body's energy. These may be respiratory changes or an awareness of blocked or low-energy areas.

Clearing — using a gentle sweeping action, the practitioner sweeps her hands over the client's body in an attempt to smooth or rebalance the client's energy field.

Intervention — the practitioner focuses her attention on specific areas of the body in order to rebalance and redirect energy.

Evaluation — the point at which the practitioner considers sufficient treatment has been given.

Therapeutic potential in nursing

Research on therapeutic touch has shown it to be effective for:

- pain relief
- anxiety
- loneliness (in the elderly)
- rehabilitation
- wound healing
- headaches
- insomnia
- hypertension
- increased haemoglobin count
- relaxation
- stress-related anxiety (see contraindications).

Clinical practice suggests it may complement care in the following:

- upper respiratory infections
- allergies
- musculoskeletal conditions
- well-being of neonates (see contraindications)
- labour and delivery (see contraindications)
- nausea
- fatigue
- comfort of the dying
- lowering temperatures
- premenstrual syndrome
- secondary, opportunistic infections of AIDS
- shingles
- the promotion of emotional and spiritual well-being.

Contraindications for use

Situations in which one must proceed with extra sensitivity and limit treatment to shorter periods are as follows:

- babies
- frail elderly
- pregnant women (particularly last trimester)
- head injuries
- emaciated patients
- psychosis
- shock.

Intentionality and centredness are the two most important qualities in a practitioner. If the practitioner is not able to become and stay centred or if they do not have the intention to help, then TT will be ineffective and the practitioner may feel drained and unwell.

Summary

Therapeutic touch is a common part of nursing practice in North America (Sayre-Adams 1993) and interest in and commitment to it has grown among nurses in the UK. TT has the potential to become integrated within mainstream nursing practice since it offers another dimension in healing and caring. Research so far suggests that TT can bring significant benefits to patients, at minimal cost. However, greater understanding of Rogers' theory as well as continued and replicated studies on TT by nurses are needed (Quinn 1989).

REFERENCES

Booth B 1993 Complementary therapy. Macmillan, London
Capra F 1976 Tao of physics. Bantam, New York
Dossey B, Keegan L, Guzzetta C, Gooding Kolkmeier L 1988 Holistic nursing: a handbook for practice. Aspen, Gaithersburg, MD
Govinda L A 1974 Foundations of Tibetan mysticism. Weiser, New York
Harvey D 1983 The power to heal: an investigation of healing and the healing experience. The Aquarian Press, London
Krieger D 1993 Accepting your power to heal. Bear, Santa Fe, NM
Kunz D 1991 The personal aura. Quest, Wheaten, IL

Therapeutic touch

161

Lutgens L R J 1991 Martha Rogers. The Science of Unitary Human Beings. Notes on nursing theories. Sage, Newbury Park, CA

Quinn J F 1988 Building a body of knowledge. Journal of Holistic Nursing 6: 37–45

Quinn J F 1989 Future directions for Therapeutic Touch research. Journal of Holistic Nursing 7: 19–25

Quinn J F 1992 Holding sacred space: the nurse as healing environment. Holistic Nursing Practice 6: 26–36

Quinn J F 1993 Psychoimmunologic effects of Therapeutic Touch on practitioners and recently bereaved recipients: a pilot study. Advances in Nursing Science 15: 13–26

Rogers M 1970 An introduction to the theoretical basis of nursing. FA Davis, Philadelphia

Sayre-Adams J 1993 Therapeutic Touch—principles and practice. Complementary Therapies in Medicine 1: 96–99

Turton P 1988 Healing: Therapeutic Touch. In: Rankin-Box D F (ed) Complementary health therapies: a guide for nurses and the caring professions. Croom Helm, Beckenham, Kent

FURTHER READING – JOURNALS

There is a large body of research on TT, much of it conducted in the US. An extended compendium of TT research can be requested from The Didsbury Trust (see Useful Addresses).

Biley F 1992 The science of unitary human beings: a contemporary literature review. Nursing Practice 15: 23–26

Heidt P R 1991 Helping patients to rest: clinical studies in Therapeutic Touch. Holistic Nursing Practice 5: 57–66

Kramer N A 1990 Comparison of Therapeutic Touch and casual touch in stress reduction of hospitalised children. Paediatric Nursing 16: 483–485

Meehan T C 1993 Therapeutic Touch and post-operative pain: a Rogerian research study. Nursing Science Quarterly 6: 69–77

Quinn J F 1984 Therapeutic Touch as energy exchange: testing the theory. Advances in Nursing Science 6: 42–49

Quinn J F 1989 Therapeutic Touch as energy exchange: replication and extension. Nursing Science Quarterly 2: 79–87

Sayre-Adams J 1994 Therapeutic Touch: a nursing function. Nursing Standard 8: 25–28

Wirth D P, Richardson J T, Eidelman W S, O'Malley A C 1993 Full thickness dermal wounds treated with non-contact Therapeutic Touch: a replication and extension. Complementary Therapies in Medicine 1: 127–132

FURTHER READING — BOOKS

Krieger D 1979 The Therapeutic Touch: how to use your hands to help or heal. Prentice Hall, Englewood Cliffs, NJ

Krieger D 1993 Accepting your power to heal. Bear, Santa Fe, NM

Macrae J 1988 Therapeutic Touch: a practical guide. Arcana, London

Meehan T C 1990 The science of unitary human beings and theory-based practice: Therapeutic Touch. In: Barrett E A M (ed) Visions of Rogers' science based nursing. National League for Nursing, New York

Rogers M E 1990 Nursing: Science of unitary irreducible human beings: update 1990. In: Barrett E A M (ed) Visions of Rogers' science based nursing. National League for Nursing, New York, p 5–11

Sayre-Adams J, Wright S 1995 Therapeutic Touch: theory and practice. Churchill Livingstone, Edinburgh (In Press)

Talbot M 1991 The holographic universe. Harper Collins, New York

USEFUL ADDRESSES

The only accredited courses in therapeutic touch are available at the Didsbury Trust, which is also the regulatory body for TT in the UK.

Didsbury Trust
Sherborne Cottage
Litton
Nr Bath BA3 4PS
Tel: 01761 241640

International Society of Rogerian Scholars
School of Nursing Studies (Mr Fran Biley)
University of Wales College of Medicine
Heath Park
Cardiff CF4 4XN
Tel: 01222 810895

Glossary

Acupuncture — derived from the Latin words *acus* (needle) and *punctara* (puncture). Chinese medical system which aims to diagnose illness and promote health by stimulating the body's self-healing powers.

Alexander technique — psychophysical postural re-education. Posture is perceived as an important contributor to health. The technique seeks to provide a process of postural re-education in order to encourage individuals to monitor consciously how they use their bodies. Thus, the technique suggests that bodily posture has an effect on physical and psychological well-being. By re-educating individuals in both posture and use of their bodies, physical and psychological well-being can be enhanced.

Aromatherapy — a form of treatment using essential oils extracted from plants which may be inhaled or massaged into the skin for therapeutic effects.

Autogenic training — a psychophysiologic form of psychotherapy, conducted by the client which involves passive concentration upon particular combinations of psychophysiological verbal stimuli. It is designed as a self-care tool.

Bach flower remedies — the use of the distilled essences of wild flowers taken diluted in water or as a lotion. The therapy is based on the premiss that disease is directly related to temperament; thus remedies treat, for example, anxiety, insomnia, disharmony.

Biofeedback — a method of training designed to enable an individual to control involuntary bodily functions, usually with the assistance of electronic equipment.

Centring — an initial stage of preparation by the practitioner in which she becomes relaxed, calm and focused on the care about to be given. This activity is described by a number of therapies, e.g. therapeutic touch and shiatsu.

Chiropractic — specializes in the diagnosis and treatment of mechanical disorders of joints and their effects on the nervous system. The spine is afforded particular attention. Displacement of spinal vertebrae may result in the manifestion of a range of seemingly unrelated symptoms. The aim of chiropractic is not to treat the symptoms but to identify the subluxation and correct it manually.

Clearing — a gentle sweeping action whereby the practitioner moves her hands over the client's body in an attempt to smooth or rebalance the energy field (see Therapeutic Touch).

Colour therapy — the use of colour in lighting, paints or materials to correct physical and psychological problems.

Counselling skills — a repertoire of learnt behaviours, both verbal and non-verbal. Adopting these skills enables a rapport to be established, facilitating the communication process.

Crystal therapy — grounded in the belief that minerals and rocks possess therapeutic forms of energy; for example, crystal creates harmony, malachite resolves inflammation.

EDR — electrodermal response, registers general levels of autonomic arousal (see Biofeedback).

Essential oil — Undiluted oil extracted from plants and commonly diluted in a carrier oil before use.

GSR — galvanic skin response, registers levels of autonomic arousal (see Biofeedback).

Hara diagnosis — a form of diagnosis used in shiatsu involving gentle palpation of the abdominal region. The focus of shiatsu is at the point on the hara known as tandem, the centre of balance and gravity.

Healing — a therapeutic form of energy exchange that may occur between two or more individuals with the conscious intention to improve health and well-being.

Herbal medicine — the use of whole plant material by trained practitioners to promote recovery from disease and to enable healing to take place.

Homoeopathy — a system of medicine based upon the Law of Similars (let like be treated with like). Effectivity is obtained by the process of dilution, in which extracts from natural sources such as plants and minerals are diluted many times in a water and alcohol base. At each dilution the mixture is vigorously shaken, a process known as succussion. It is this process which homoeopaths believe initiates the healing potency of the dilution.

Humour and laughter therapy — a humorous or amusing intervention used by the health care professional or patient and designed to be of benefit to the patient.

Hypnosis — in health care, the deliberate use of the trance state to enhance the sense of health and well-being.

Iridology — a diagnostic tool based on the assumption that the iris can indicate the general status of internal organs. Iridology may be used by herbalists and naturopaths.

Kinesiology — a therapy that tests different muscles to identify and/or prevent allergies.

Massage — the conscious, deliberate and often formalized use of the instinctive response to comfort another person by touch.

Meridians — conceptual channels along which Qi energy flows in the body (see Acupuncture and Shiatsu).

Nutritional therapy — based on the assumption that the state of one's health is directly contingent upon what is eaten. Nutritional therapy focuses upon the effects certain foods have on health and well-being.

Osteopathy — manipulation of joints and spinal vertebrae directed towards resolving mechanical problems of the body. Thus abnormal tension in muscles and ligaments can be relieved and self-healing facilitated.

Placebo response — a self-healing response.

Process of counselling — occurs within a non-directive therapeutic relationship, whereby the client will be enabled to self-actualize and develop his own abilities to resolve or accept his situation.

Radionics — based on the concept that each part of the body vibrates at specific rates. In illness the vibrations alter. Changes can be corrected with instruments that send back energy to the affected organs. Treatment can be done using blood or hair samples without the presence of the client.

Reflexology — a treatment which applies varying degrees of pressure to different parts of the body, commonly the hands and feet in order to promote health and well-being. It is suggested that there are reflexes or zones running along the body and terminating in the hands or feet. All systems and organs are said to be reflected on to the hands or feet and by applying gentle pressure to specific areas of the hands or feet a change can be effected elsewhere in the body.

Relaxation — a state of consciousness characterized by feelings of peace and release from tension, anxiety and fear.

Shiatsu — literally means 'finger pressure'. A hands-on therapy which works on the energetic pathways to balance and strengthen the body in order to facilitate self-healing.

Succussion — used in homoeopathy, a process whereby natural diluted substances are vigorously shaken. Homoeopaths believe that it is this process that facilitates the healing potential of the dilution.

Target organ — term used in biofeedback to describe the organ or part of the body from which changing levels of activity can be demonstrated, for example skin, brain, heart.

Therapeutic touch (TT) — described as an energy field interaction between two or more people with the intention to rebalance or repattern the energy field in order to facilitate relaxation and self-healing.

Trance — an altered state of consciousness.

Visualization — the technique of using the imagination to create any desired changes in an individual's life.

Yin/Yang — represents the dynamic balance of energy. Yang energy is characterized by heat, movement, activity and excess; Yin energy relates more to cold, sluggishness, inactivity and deficiency. A balance of each kind of energy is necessary for health.

Zones — a term used in reflexology. It is suggested that the body's innate energy flows through reflexes or zones which terminate in the hands or feet.

Additional addresses

Alexander technique

Society of Teachers of the
Alexander Technique (STAT)
20 London House
266 Fulham road
London SW10 9EL
Tel: 0171 351 0828

Alexander Technique Teaching
Centre
188 Old Street
London EC1V 9BP

Chiropractic

British Chiropractic Association
29 Whitley Street
Reading
Berkshire RG2 OEG
Tel: 01734 757 557

Scottish Chiropractic Association
12 Walker Street
Edinburgh 3
Scotland
Tel: 0131 225 7743

Osteopathy

General Council and Register of
Osteopaths
56 London Street
Reading
Berks RG1 4SQ

British College of Naturopathy
and Osteopathy
6 Netherall Gardens
London NW3 5RR

Natural Therapeutic and
Osteopathic Society and Register
168 High street
Maldon
Essex CM2 7BX
Tel: 01621 859094

Cranial Osteopathic Association
478 Baker Street
Enfield
Middlesex EN1 3QS
Tel: 0181 367 5561

Research and education sources

Centre for Complementary
Medicine North West
School of Nursing and Health
Studies
Stockport College of Further and
Higher Education North West
Wellington Road South
Stockport SK1 3UQ
Tel: 0161 958 3561

Complementary Therapies Forum
Royal College of Nursing (RCN)
20 Cavendish Square
London W1M OAB
Tel: 0171 409 3333

Research Council for
Complementary Medicine (RCCM)
5th floor
60 Great Ormond Street
London WC1 3JF
Tel: 0171 833 8897

Medical Research Council
20 Park Crescent
London W1N 4AL
Tel: 0171 636 5422

Institute for Complementary
Medicine
PO Box 194
London SE16 1QZ
Tel: 0171 237 5165

Centre for the Study of
Complementary Medicine
51 Bedford Place
Southampton
Hampshire
SO1 2DG
Tel: 01703 334752

Confederation of Healing
Organizations
The Red and White House
113 High Street
Berkhampstead
Hertfordshire HP4 2DJ
Tel: 01442 870660

INDEX

Index

173

Index

177

Notes